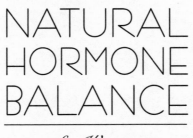

NATURAL
HORMONE
BALANCE

for Women

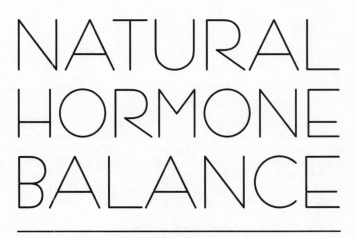

NATURAL HORMONE BALANCE

for Women

Look Younger, Feel Stronger,
and Live Life with Exuberance

UZZI REISS, M.D./OB.-GYN.

with Martin Zucker

POCKET BOOKS

NEW YORK   LONDON   TORONTO   SYDNEY   SINGAPORE

The ideas, procedures, and suggestions in this book are not intended as a substitute for the medical advice of your trained health professional. All matters regarding your health require medical supervision. Consult your physician before adoping the suggestions in this book, as well as about any condition that may require diagnosis or medical attention. The author and publisher disclaim any liability arising directly or indirectly from the use of the book.

POCKET BOOKS, a division of Simon & Schuster, Inc.
1230 Avenue of the Americas, New York, NY 10020

Library of Congress Cataloging-in-Publication Data

Reiss, Uzzi.
    Natural hormone balance for women : look younger, feel stronger, and live life with exuberance /
Uzzi Reiss and Martin Zucker.
        p. cm.
    Includes bibliographical references.
    ISBN 0-7434-0665-6
    1. Rejuvenation. 2. Aging—Prevention. 3. Hormones—Therapeutic use. 4. Longevity.
5. Health. I. Zucker, Martin. II. Title.

RA776.75.R45 2001
615'.36'082—dc21   00-049139

First Pocket Books hardcover printing January 2001

10   9   8   7   6   5   4   3   2

POCKET and colophon are registered trademarks of
Simon & Schuster, Inc.

Designed by Alma Orenstein

Printed in the U.S.A.

To all my patients who have taught me so much; to Yael, my beloved companion and advisor for thirty years; and to my children, Yfat, Jacob, and Itay.

—UZZI REISS

Once again to Rosita, my soul mate.

—MARTIN ZUCKER

Note to the Reader

This book about the use of natural hormones is not intended as medical advice and should not be used to replace medical care or any therapeutic program recommended by a physician. It is meant for information and education only.

If you have symptoms or suffer from an illness, you should consult with an appropriate health professional for your condition.

If you are currently taking prescription drugs, do not discontinue them or replace them based on any of the information or recommendations appearing in this book without first consulting your doctor.

Clinical experience indicates that natural hormones do not interfere with medication. However, if you are under treatment for any condition and are considering taking natural hormones, we recommend you first inform your physician and obtain his or her opinion.

Contents

PART FOUR
Building on the Basics: Using Other Natural Hormones to Stay Younger, More Vital, and Healthier

PART FIVE
Putting It All Together

Appendices

Foreword

by Jesse Lynn Hanley, M.D., co-author of *What Your Doctor May Not Tell You About Premenopause: Balance Your Hormones and Your Life from Thirty to Fifty* (Warner Books)

Hormones. It's a subject that has women confused and fearful.

As a physician who practices wellness-oriented health care and has been using natural hormones, I predict that the book you are about to read will banish that confusion and fear and exert a major influence for many years to come. It provides a fresh opportunity to raise the level of women's health to the maximum.

This book is about knowledge—detailed, practical, how-to knowledge that is urgently needed. With this knowledge, you—and women everywhere—have the potential to demystify the often-puzzling hormonal cycles and restore balance to your body.

Today, women are very interested in natural hormones and are looking for answers from their physicians. This book provides those answers.

Women want to know if natural hormones are safe. They are as safe as our own hormones and certainly safer than synthetic hormones. This book gives you guidelines for using them wisely and effectively. I know from my own medical practice, where I have prescribed natural hormones for more than a dozen years, that they are the safest and most effective option available to women.

The question that really must be asked is whether the *pharmaceutical* hormones routinely prescribed to women are safe. These are hormone formulations often extracted from horses or concocted in test tubes. Can they possibly be safer than natural hormones that are exact replicas of what a woman's own body makes? I don't think so. Research, in fact, shows that pharmaceutical hormones can have very disturbing side effects. Just read the *Physician's Desk Reference (PDR)!*

Doctors who have not used natural hormones often question how well they are absorbed in the body. This issue really goes beyond hormones to the fact that each of us is an individual, reacting differently to all that we take into our bodies—hormones, medicines, remedies, and even food. If you and I each were to take a hormone pill with the same dosage, you might absorb five times the amount that I would. The quantity you absorb might be fine for you, and the amount I absorb fine for me. That's individuality.

Uzzi Reiss goes to great length in this book to explain the importance of individuality. He explains in detail how to recognize your individual reactions to natural hormones, whether you take them in a pill, sublingual drops, or a gel applied to your skin. His careful, step-by-step instructions raise the practical value of this book above that of all others. He tells you what you need to know first and foremost: how to interpret your individual reactions and how to adjust your own hormone intake accordingly for maximum benefit.

Dr. Reiss's book is a landmark reference, packed with the revelations of twenty years of clinical experience, patient feedback, and mounting scientific research. It brings the knowledge of natural hormone usage a quantum leap forward—for both the female patient and her doctor.

This book also covers such important issues as nutrition and stress, which are frequently neglected when women are counseled about their health. Dr. Reiss discusses certain supplements that he has found extremely beneficial for patients and supportive of hormonal therapy. He also expresses concern over the current calcium mania, which can contribute to a deficiency in another mineral important for female health, magnesium. The book also addresses the overlooked but critical topic of environmental chemicals and how they can poison our food, health, and hormonal balance.

Dr. Reiss writes in depth about breast cancer, a condition very close to my heart—both my mother and sister died of this disease. Significantly, he makes a strong argument for the use of natural progesterone in preventing breast cancer. I use natural progesterone myself for this purpose. It may be the single most powerful agent at a woman's disposal that is also simple, appropriate, and doesn't require lifestyle changes. This is vital information for women, because our own production of the hormone often declines well before menopause, leaving us without a critical element of natural protection. We used to think that the decline of estrogen before menopause caused all our problems and changes, and that the solution was to take only estrogen. Now we are realizing that for many women the drop in progesterone may be an even greater source of risks and problems. By replacing progesterone, we are restoring balance and regaining lost protection.

Many of the hormones described in the book require a prescription. Show this book to your gynecologist or family physician, and encourage her or him to read it. Nowadays, a good deal of postgraduate education is coming to doctors via their patients. And, increasingly, physicians are responding to their patients' interest in natural healing. If your physician shows no interest in natural hormones, you may want to seek out another health professional who is familiar with them to serve as your health care partner. We are all unique, and we all need a little help with this new approach. In my experience, the benefits of natural hormones are so great that it is well worth the effort to find an open-minded, experienced, and interested professional. This book tells you how to find such professionals in your area and how to monitor your progress with them.

Uzzi Reiss is my gynecologist, and the gynecologist for many of my patients. From teenagers to menopausal women, he has helped us balance our hormone-based female problems and taught us to attain a higher level of health. This book is a transcription of his experience with thousands of patients and can help grandmothers, mothers, and daughters alike.

Yes, Dr. Reiss is a man giving advice to women. Yet his respect for women and concern for women's health has made him a champion of women's rights. He is the most caring, kind, and loving gynecologist I know—male or female—practicing in the greater Los Angeles area. I am sure that as you read his book and absorb the great detail he provides to help you understand and obtain maximum benefit from natural hormones, you will also sense his caring nature. For so many years, Dr. Reiss has been the only gynecologist I know who is steadfastly committed to natural hormones as the wiser, safer, and better option. To anybody who questions that, he answers, How can you possibly think that something artificial is better for us than what our body makes?

This book is all about this wiser, safer, and better option.

Introduction

Taking Hormones without Worry

During more than twenty years as a gynecologist I have treated thousands of women, from down-and-out individuals at free clinics in the Bronx to the most wealthy and famous at my Beverly Hills practice. Rich or poor, they usually have one thing in common: *a great desire to stay youthful and healthy.*

In past times, most women gave birth to many children, labored for decades to raise them, and lived much shorter lives. For them, the idea of rejuvenation was irrelevant.

For the modern woman, life is a whole new game.

From an evolutionary perspective, the female was designed for multiple cycles of pregnancy and breast-feeding. This was nature's way of preserving the species. Up until the time of modern hygiene and medicine, most offspring never reached reproductive age. They fell victim to infectious diseases, lack of sanitation, and an ever-perilous environment.

The modern woman has broken from the historic pattern of multiple pregnancies. She often delays the onset of reproduction. She has fewer children or doesn't become pregnant at all. She takes birth control pills. She is exposed to an unprecedented array of environmental chemicals, processed food, and career opportunities.

The new reality has brought overdue choices and liberation, but with a price: hormonal chaos, increased risk of disease and so-called female problems, and accelerated aging. This is meant not as a criticism but as an observation based on treating more than ten thousand women.

Patients come to me not only for relief of their gynecological problems, but also increasingly to solve their hormonal chaos, restore balance, *and achieve the highest possible level of health.* They want to infuse zest and youthfulness into the aging process.

Shortly after starting my medical practice I learned about *natural* hormones—first progesterone, then estrogen, and then others. I found them to be an exciting, safe, and effective way to help patients accomplish their health goals and also reduce the need for medical drugs and surgery.

A woman who feels good, sleeps well, has balanced moods, and a healthy sex drive may tend to believe that hormones are unnecessary for her. She may be right. However, she may also be missing a potentially huge amount of added vigor and youthfulness.

Many of my first-time patients simply don't feel good. They don't sleep well. The may experience hot flashes or roller-coaster moods they can't seem to control. They may have menstrual problems, or their sex drive isn't what they would like it to be.

Often they come in desperation. Nothing has worked for them. They may follow a healthy lifestyle, eat the right foods, take supplements, and exercise. They may even meditate or follow a spiritual path. Yet they complain about their health and looks.

I typically encounter fear and confusion when I bring up the subject of hormones for the first time. It is rare, in fact, if a woman is not fearful or confused. Every patient seems to have her own hormone story or knows someone who experienced side effects from hormones. Many know women who have died from breast cancer.

"I've heard such horror stories from friends," a typical new patient will tell me. "They have trouble with their cycles. They gain weight. They have irregular bleeding. Everything got *worse* after they started on hormones. And I hear all these medical reports about hormones and breast cancer."

Let's look at the truths and myths behind the fear.

Hormonal Misinformation

Most women, like my new patients, are fearful and confused about aging and hormones. Much of my practice involves taking time to reassure patients that their hormones are not going to kill them.

No wonder that women are fearful and confused. They are subjected to a constant bombardment of misinformation about the dangers of female hormones. As a gynecologist who sees how the minds and souls of women are seriously disturbed by the distortions, my blood boils.

During one particular week while writing this book, a major medical journal published a study announcing yet again to women that hormones increase the risk of breast cancer. The study was widely reported throughout the media.

"Study links breast cancer, hormone use," the *Los Angeles Times* proclaimed on page one.

"Menopause complications using 2 hormones to protect bones and heart add to cancer risk," warned *USA Today*.

A similar study from a West Coast medical center followed a few days later and was also given prominent exposure in the media.

Undoubtedly you are aware of these and similar reports linking hormones to cancer and other problems. Such reports have been coming out for years.

If I were a woman, I would be paranoid about my own hormones. I would be especially confused if I were perimenopausal or menopausal, when women most dramatically feel the symptoms of changing hormones in their bodies.

I might begin viewing my breasts as time bombs set to explode with cancer and kill me.

I might begin to think that my ovaries could just as easily end my life as create new life.

I would wonder: should I remove my breasts? Then I won't die from breast cancer.

Should I remove my ovaries early? Then they won't produce cancer-causing estrogen.

What if I want to have children? That's no problem. They have miraculous fertilization techniques.

And what if my doctor prescribes hormonal replacement therapy? Should I run out the door?

New patients tell me things like this every day. For many women the word *hormone* has become synonymous with cancer, death, and the beginning of the end of life.

What the News Reports Don't Tell You

Something is very wrong about medical reports indicating that your female hormones can kill you. These are the same hormones that make you a woman, that keep your breasts full and your skin young, that prepare the womb and nurture the growing fetus. Your wrinkles, your fragile bones, your drooping breasts, and your waning sensuality are due to the loss of these same hormones as you age.

What's wrong with the medical reports and the way they are translated to you is that you are not being told one simple fact: *there is nothing in common between the hormones produced in your body and the "hormones" involved in these reports.*

If I mention the word *tail*, would you associate it with a human being? If I mention *hay*, would you associate it with a brunch in a restaurant?

Similarly, the estrogen "hormone" used in these studies is not your human female estrogen hormone. It is a patented, chemicalized hormonal substitute—a drug. It is usually Premarin or some similar compound based on the estrogen found in the urine of pregnant horses.

Likewise, the widely prescribed "progestins" that are the subject of the medical reports and studies you hear about may have names sounding similar to your own progesterone. But progestins are drugs like Provera, and they are not the same as your own progesterone.

During the evolution of the human species prior to the advent of patented, chemicalized hormonal substitutes, a woman's body was never exposed to such substances. For sure, there are problems with them.

Knowing the difference between chemicalized, hormonal substitutes and natural hormones can also open your horizon to the exciting new frontier of natural hormone replacement and supplementation.

I do not recommend patented, chemicalized hormonal substitutes to patients. Instead, I emphasize natural hormones that are *precise replicas of your own hormones.* I use them to prolong the optimum hormonal balance that women have in their twenties and thirties, and the results are magnificent.

I tell patients not to be afraid, because these natural hormones are fundamental to the way the body operates and are identical copies of what the body produces.

The structure of a house includes a roof, a frame, walls, and a foundation. You may come to me and tell me that you are buying new furniture, repainting your house, and making your residence more resistant to the elements. You may be remodeling it, giving it a "face-lift," so to speak.

But what about the foundation, the basis on which everything rests? The topside may get a face-lift and new paint, but the foundation underneath may be cracking and deteriorating relentlessly with time. Every day it crumbles a bit more. Hormones are like the foundation. They decrease in your body with

The medical reports are not about your own hormones. They are about patented, chemicalized hormonal substitutes. Knowing that difference can set you free from confusion and fear.

age. But there are things you can do to slow down the deterioration this loss produces.

But wait, you may be thinking, hormone replacement is a new idea. It hasn't been practiced throughout history. If it wasn't needed or used in the past, why should we use it now? Why should I consider aging an unnatural process?

In a 1995 *Time* magazine article on hormones, Duke University gynecologist Charles Hammond, M.D., noted that "as women have lived increasingly longer lives, they are facing problems their grandmothers never faced. At the turn of the century, women died soon after their ovaries quit."

In history, humans never lived as long as we do, but they also never went through such prolonged deterioration and slow death. If you have seen your elderly parents or a loved one deteriorate, you surely don't want to think about the same thing happening to you. But we will all decline and lose our vitality. Only a few are so genetically blessed to be able to go the distance erect and vital.

You can paint your house as many times as you want. You can remodel it every five years. You can have multiple face-lifts. But the foundation still crumbles underneath. My message is not to forget the foundation but to preserve it.

"Try natural hormones," I will tell a patient. "They will help preserve your foundation and give you longer-lasting support to the rest of the unique structure that is you."

"But maybe I'll take too much of a hormone and feel worse from the side effects," the patient may answer.

"Well," I try to reassure her, "you take vitamin E every day and do you know if it is helping you or not? Do you know if you are taking enough or too much? With natural hormones, you will always know. When you take more than you need, your body will let you know. And that's what I will teach you—how to recognize the signs. When your body speaks, that will be your cue. You will simply have passed your tolerance at that particular time."

I have always learned from my patients. Their feedback has enabled me to help them become masters in the use of natural hormones at any stage of life, whether they are young women out of hormonal balance or older women negotiating a particularly rocky road during early menopause.

Now I wish to share this experience and help make masters of women everywhere, of all ages, women who are interested in improving their health, reducing the symptoms associated with the aging process, and slowing down their biological clocks.

The Benefits of Natural Hormones

The positive experiences of thousands of patients over the years have clearly demonstrated the effectiveness and safety of natural hormones. The feedback has enabled me to create the step-by-step program for safe and optimum hormonal balance you will find in this book.

Please keep in mind that I am not a researcher. I am not a scientist. I am a clinician who observes closely the outcome of treatments. If they don't work, I don't use them. Natural hormones have worked magnificently for my patients and produced multiple benefits. Here's a short list of them:

- More energy and stamina.
- Less confusion and "foggy mind."
- Better memory.
- PMS symptoms reduced or eliminated.
- Menopause symptoms reduced or eliminated.
- Healthier and more youthful skin.
- Balanced moods and fewer mood swings.
- Normalization of weight.
- Less depression.
- Less anxiety.
- Better muscle definition.
- Better sleep.
- Enhanced sexuality.

These same benefits are available to you through my program of natural hormones. In this book I will teach you, as I have taught my patients, the following:

- How to use natural hormones safely for maximum effect.
- When to use them . . . and when not to use them.
- The differences between patented, chemicalized hormonal substitutes (what all the confusing news reports are about) and natural hormones.
- What forms of natural hormones are the best for you in your situation—pills, gels, drops, or creams.
- The possible responses you will feel from each hormone.
- How to monitor your responses and adjust your individual dosage for maximum results.
- How to work with your physician to monitor your progress with objective medical tests.

In regard to the last point let me make one thing clear: *no book, doctor, Nobel Prize winner, or anybody else on earth but you alone can determine your optimum hormonal balance.* I will provide the information to guide you, just as I do for my own patients. I can't tell them, or you, what is the precise optimum level. Each of you is an individual with individual tolerances and requirements.

This book is not a scientific journey into the complex molecular and cellular world of hormones. *It is a manual, a practical guide for using natural hormones safely and without worry and adjusting them to match your individual needs and goals.* The book is a partnership.

I give you the information. You take the action. You become the master of your hormonal destiny. You reap the dividends of better health and the preservation of youthfulness.

This book is intended for women of all ages—the young, the middle-aged, and the elderly. For mothers, grandmothers, and granddaughters.

Can it help all of you? I don't think so. But it should help most of you. There will always be a few people who do not respond, whose conditions are very complex, and who require highly individualized treatment with a skilled physician. I see many patients like this in my practice, some of whom are extremely difficult to treat.

As a clinical doctor, I have made it a priority to consider the individuality of each patient. No two patients are the same. No two readers are the same. Identical twins with the same condition may require totally different approaches. There is no single medication, no single dosage, for each and every person. When we investigate the causes of problems and treat the individual and not the disease, we are much better able to help patients. This is the way we as physicians can decrease the unacceptably high incidence of chronic disease and drug-related illnesses and side effects, as well as create a healthier society.

The treatments I develop for my patients are designed to fit into each lifestyle and each patient's ability to follow through. Because you are not my patient, I cannot customize a program to fit your situation. Therefore I have included detailed guidelines in this book to cover menopause, peri-menopause, and a woman's younger years. With these guidelines you will be able to individualize a program to meet your own situation.

The book is not intended to convince you to use a natural hormone replacement program. From a strict medical standpoint, the only time that a woman *needs* hormone replacement is when her body is overwhelmed by estrogen and she doesn't have enough progesterone. Estrogen dominance can lead to endometrial cancer, endometriosis, fibroids, and abnormal bleeding, and needs to be counteracted with progesterone replacement.

Other than this use, hormone replacement is purely elective. It is for people, like many of my patients, who want to restore or prolong their healthfulness and youthfulness. If you are an individual who is not content to allow your antiaging hormones to run down with the relentless ticking of your biological clock, this book is for you.

My patients want to take control of their bodies and responsibility for their health. They want to learn what makes their biological clocks tick and work with me to make individualized adjustments. We fine-tune the process for maximum effects.

I see many patients who have no physical, mental, or sexual problems, and yet take one or more of the hormones discussed in this book. They adjust the hormones to their body. Most feel significantly better. Others may not feel any difference immediately but continue to take the hormones with the goal of enhancing long-term health and enabling the body to operate longer at maximum capacity.

Some patients tell me that they never knew they had a hormonal deficiency, yet they never really felt entirely well until they started this program. Natural hormones can resolve many symptoms.

Whatever condition or goal brings these patients to me, the great majority soar on the program. You can do the same.

How to Use This Book

I have organized this book as a *one-stop* resource for understanding and using natural hormones. It is a very doable program.

I advise you first to read through the book. Learn exactly what are the physical and emotional expressions of different hormonal deficiencies. As you read you will come across the issues and symptoms that most concern you. Afterward, you can refer back to those points of personal interest and follow the guidelines for hormonal use.

I have put great emphasis on estrogen and progesterone, the hormones of prime concern to women. These hormones generally need the most attention because each woman has a totally different response and requirement. These responses and requirements change with the way the hormones fluctuate in the body. Sooner or later, you will be deficient in estrogen and progesterone, and you will face the decision: whether or not to replace them.

You may first want to learn to balance estrogen and progesterone and then perhaps add other natural hormones. You may not think you need or want to supplement other hormones, but still it will help you to read the information and see what the options and benefits are.

In part one I will discuss the difference between natural and chemicalized hormones. I will also cover the issue of individuality, because it is so important to using hormones successfully. Fixed amounts of hormones, or even prescription drugs or vitamins, don't work for everybody. We are all individuals.

Also up front is a strong message to pay attention to your stress and blood sugar levels. These factors have a major impact on hormonal health and your ability to achieve optimum balance.

Part two focuses on estrogen, the essence of femininity. The chapters in this section discuss how to use natural estrogen for menopause and perimenopause and how it can help certain younger women who are estrogen deficient.

In part three I turn to progesterone, the great hormonal harmonizer for women. I will instruct you how to use progesterone for different conditions and stages of life, including its powerful effect against PMS.

Next, in part four, I cover other hormones that can make major improvements to the quality of your life. These hormones are testosterone, human growth hormone, DHEA, melatonin, and pregnenolone. I will teach you how to put these natural hormones to use safely for antiaging and gynecological benefits.

Finally, in the last part of the book, I will explain how to combine hormones for maximum effect. In this section I will also address the complicated issue of breast cancer and hormones. By reading this chapter you will learn that hormone replacement is really a woman's best friend and protector.

In this book, I do not cover thyroid hormone in depth. Thyroid is a major consideration by itself, and there are already good books available on the subject.

As you embark on this self-improvement journey, be sure to keep your physician informed. Besides personal interest in your health status, your doctor can perform the periodic tests and monitoring necessary to keep track of important hormonal balances and biochemical activities in your body. Chapter 4 discusses how to make your physician a partner in your natural hormone program.

I invite you now to embark on an exciting exploration of antiaging possibilities with me. A "natural hormone revolution" lies ahead, and someday soon replacement with natural hormones will be as commonplace as taking nutritional supplements.

PART ONE

The Promise of Natural Hormone Replacement

1

Why Natural Hormones?

> There is nothing mysterious about aging. Aging is simply an inherited hormonal, neuroendocrine program . . . that can be modified, delayed or even reversed.
>
> —WALTER PIERPAOLI, M.D.

For two years, Carole had been gaining weight and experiencing abnormal periods and breast tenderness. She had become increasingly nervous. Her premenstrual mood swings were causing strains in her relationships.

Now, at forty-five, she had had enough. She decided to overcome her problems with aggressive lifestyle changes.

She hired a personal trainer and began a vigorous exercise program.

She hired a personal nutritionist and went on a special diet and supplement program.

She started yoga.

Carole's efforts gave her some relief, but not enough. Frustrated, she went to her physician, who offered her a birth control pill.

"This will rebalance you," her doctor said.

What Carole experienced was anything but rebalance.

Her weight ballooned. Her mood swings became worse. She lost her sex drive. The only regularity she achieved was an artificially normal cycle. Yet during the week of the cycle that she used the birth control placebo, she had migraines, couldn't sleep well, and started to have hot flashes.

Fed up, she stopped taking the pill. Within six months, her anxiety decreased, her moods swings lessened, and her weight dropped. Now, however, she was depressed.

"I don't enjoy waking up anymore and seeing the sun and look forward to what the day brings," she told me as she sat in my office during her first appointment. "I don't feel like going out and showing myself to the world."

Carole (not her real name) is an established actress. The constant changes in her body and outlook were affecting both her personal and professional life.

"Before I was showered with scripts and had my choice of roles," she said. "That's changed. Because I've changed so much. No one seems to want to audition me. I'm not the same person anymore. Some people think I am on drugs."

Carole's story was a variation on a theme I have heard many times. Initially, her body was overproducing estrogen and not producing enough progesterone. The birth control pill was the wrong choice for the wrong person. It accentuated the excess estrogen and aggravated the progesterone deficiency. When she stopped the pill—and its payload of chemicalized hormones—her own hormones had taken a new shift and she was in a different state. Her estrogen level had fallen significantly and her progesterone was lower than before. She showed classic signs of estrogen deficiency, even though she wasn't in menopause. Her estrogen level, rising and falling like a roller coaster, was still within the boundaries of the so-called normal range. Yet she would certainly ride that roller coaster right into menopause.

What she needed was a way to restore her lost stability and with the same hormone—estrogen—that had given her stability for many years.

I instructed Carole how to use natural estrogen, how to increase her dosage when she experienced signs of deficiency, and how to decrease on those days when her body produced more.

She went from being a woman whose hormones were controlling her and undermining her life to being a woman fully in control, and enjoying renewed vigor, clarity, and health.

Carole had been a victim of rigid medical thinking that too often fails to see beyond "normal range" blood tests and recognize the real turmoil that hormonal fluctuations and shifts can generate in a woman's body. Carole took control of her hormones and took control of her life.

* * *

Hormones are molecules that serve as messengers in an amazing system of inner intelligence that organizes your physiology. Life itself is based on this inner intelligence.

There are countless hormones generated within the body, many of which we don't yet clearly understand. They are secreted by glands—such as the adrenals, ovaries, and thyroid—that are governed by higher centers in the brain.

The hormones travel through your bloodstream in a communication network that links the higher centers of your brain to the DNA command posts operating in the several hundred trillion cells of your adult body.

On outer and inner membranes of the cells are receptor sites that function like locks on a door. In order to get in and tell the DNA what to do, you need the right key, and hormones are the keys. They travel to specific target cells, unlock the receptor sites, and deliver their biochemical message for processing. They turn on or turn off specific cellular functions, and measure cellular activity throughout the system.

As scientists probe deeper and deeper into the labyrinths of this molecular world and learn more about its countless parts and partnerships, the complexities of the system become more and more wondrous. The more we learn, the more we realize we don't know.

We do know, however, that the glands produce greater or lesser amounts of different hormones at different times of the day, month, and stage of life, and according to your activities. And we do know that nearly all of them start to decline after we reach our midtwenties.

This book is concerned about the rise and fall of major hormones that are of primary concern to women—estrogen, progesterone, testosterone, mela-

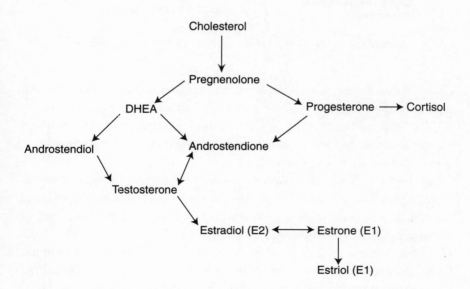

SEQUENCE OF SELECTED HORMONE PRODUCTION IN THE BODY

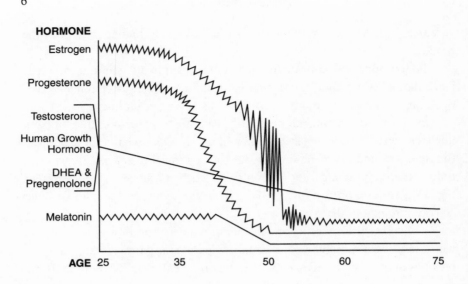

HORMONE

Estrogen

Progesterone

Testosterone

Human Growth
Hormone

DHEA &
Pregnenolone

Melatonin

AGE 25   35   50   60   75

AGE-RELATED DECLINE OF HORMONES

Estrogen: 30% drop by age 50, then sharp drop with fluctuations in menopause.

Progesterone: 75% loss from age 35 to 50, then continuing decline.

Human Growth Hormone, DHEA, Pregnenolone, Testosterone: 50% loss from age 25 to 50, followed by an additional 50% loss by age 75.

Melatonin: Small decline from age 25 to 40, followed by sharp drop.

tonin, DHEA, human growth hormone, and pregnenolone—and how natural replicas of these hormones can be used for health and antiaging benefits.

Yes, I did say testosterone. You might think of testosterone as something exclusively male, but female ovaries manufacture it as well for purposes that are very important to a woman.

In this book, you will learn how to use these pivotal hormones for personal improvements. You will learn to take control of them instead of being controlled by their fluctuations. You will learn to direct your hormones just as a conductor directs a symphony.

I often tell my patients to think in terms of a symphony of hormones. Each hormone produces a particular effect that contributes to the overall function of the physiology, just as individual instruments produce specific effects that contribute to the overall sound of a symphony.

No symphony can produce its majestic sound without a conductor, and hormones themselves cannot produce a beautiful melody of health if there is no conductor on duty. You are the conductor. You have the ability to control your hormones so that the "music" they make is sweet: hormonal balance and well-being.

Many women today are never in hormonal balance—at any age. A woman who is hormonally imbalanced at twenty-five usually continues that way through perimenopause and menopause unless she gets proper help.

For many women, *unhealthy aging is primarily a hormonal issue.* The day they begin to deteriorate is the day their hormones start declining from a peak level. For some it is earlier, for others later.

I encourage my patients not to wait until they reach hormonal ground zero before taking action. An antiaging strategy has the potential to powerfully offset and delay the negative effects of hormonal decline on function and appearance. The deficits that take place within the body are often irreversible if you wait too long. For instance, wrinkling: you will probably not be able to significantly reverse the presence of serious wrinkling by using natural hormones, but you can significantly slow down the wrinkling process.

Some of my patients use all the hormones I will describe in this book; some use only one or two. Some start with one and then add another later for a specific need. After I make my recommendations, the options are up to each individual patient.

As I discuss each hormone, I will spell out its potential for relief of symptoms, better health, and antiaging benefits. I encourage you to take that information and measure it against what is going on in your body and what your individual health and antiaging goals are.

If a fifty-year-old woman sees her physician and complains of losing half the movement in her pinky finger, she will receive serious medical attention: prescriptions, X rays, perhaps an MRI. She will be referred to a hand specialist and perhaps undergo surgery.

This same woman has probably already lost half of her hormone production. She sits in front of the mirror and asks why she looks and feels like she does. The decline of hormones inside her body affects how she looks and feels, and also affects countless aspects of her physiology. If she complains of lost hormones, she will likely be told that it's natural to age, slow down, wrinkle, and lose sexuality. She might not be encouraged to start with hormones and certainly not replace the full range of falling hormones in her body.

But the availability of natural hormones makes this argument obsolete.

The Fountain of Youthfulness

Replenishing and balancing hormones reinfuses health—and youthfulness— into the aging process. *It is a primary way to repair damage of the past, alleviate present symptoms, and redirect the body into a healthier mode for a more vital future.* Because the role of hormones is so central, realigning them strengthens the entire physiology and all its systems.

This process is not a fountain of youth, but it is a fountain of youthfulness. We can never really be as we were at age twenty-five, but we can fine-tune and retool our internal machinery through natural hormones and other non-invasive methods. We can re-create health and longevity to the fullest level that our genetic programming allows. This is where hormonal replacement therapy and antiaging medicine merge.

The marvels of modern medicine have truly helped to extend life span, yet they haven't solved the problems of chronic disease. Nor have they really enhanced the quality of longer life. For many people, living longer lives than in the past involves a drawn-out ordeal. For them, there are no golden years, only years of rust. Natural hormonal replacement is a way to accentuate the gold and minimize the rust.

Preventive medicine has helped combat many diseases of aging. As the new field of antiaging medicine has emerged, researchers and practitioners have come together to prolong life and enhance its quality. Experts in physiology, biology, and biochemistry are sharing their findings with antiaging specialists who are applying the research to their patients.

Antiaging medicine seeks to correct the decline of important age-related conditions. It also attempts to identify and arrest the initial physiological changes that cause accelerated aging or turn the body from healthy to unhealthy functioning. Those of us who practice antiaging medicine study and utilize nutritional and hormonal factors to accomplish these goals.

Not everyone will be interested in the antiaging aspects of natural hormones. Many may choose to use them for specific needs—improving memory, becoming stronger, increasing energy, sleeping better, or overcoming gynecological disorders. As you will see, natural hormones work particularly well for all these concerns.

I have also seen natural hormones work effectively for many younger women whose own hormone levels are too high or too low. Such extremes can create many problems, but a touch of natural estrogen can put life back into a young woman with too little estrogen who is tall, flat-chested, and subtly depressed. Natural progesterone can help a young woman with an irregular cycle, heavy bleeding, severe breast pain, and water retention.

All of these possible benefits of natural hormones will be covered in this book. Young or old, the use of natural hormones represents an important advancement in our ability to optimize and protect our biological assets.

So What Exactly Are Natural Hormones?

Women are reading and hearing a lot about natural hormones these days. In fact, they are bombarded from all sides with information. New patients often say they have tried to make sense of it all but are confused. Many who look to the Internet for answers come away even more confused by the sheer volume of marketing hype. Women are being told they can replace hormones, but nobody is telling them how to do it on an individual basis.

Increasingly women ask their physicians for guidance, but most physicians don't have the answers or the experience with natural hormones. *The prescriptions that physicians have written for years are largely patented, chemicalized hormonal substitutes. These products are not exact replicas of what you have in your body, and you will not be able to achieve optimum individual balance with them.*

In recent years, natural hormone replacements have become widely available to women. What distinguishes these natural hormones is that they are exact replicas—not just similar—to the hormones in the body. This is what makes them natural. This is also what makes them preferable to the chemicalized hormonal substitutes that provide reassurance and relief for some, and fear and side effects for others.

According to a study conducted at South Dakota State University's College of Pharmacy, an estimated 2.01 million visits for medication-related problems were made to physicians in the United States during 1995. Such visits were greater among women. The leading therapeutic agents responsible for these visits were synthetic hormone substitutes (13.32 percent), followed by antibiotics (11.5 percent).

Many women don't take the hormones prescribed for them. They simply stop taking them after a while because of the side effects or stop because of the scare about hormones and breast cancer. In chapter 24, I will share some reassuring news with you: *the scientific evidence overwhelmingly shows that estrogen hormonal prescriptions do not increase your risk of dying from breast cancer, and in fact, reduce the risk of fatal breast cancer.*

The problem with most of the conventional substitutes commonly prescribed to women is that they are different in chemical structure from the hormones that your body produces. This difference aggravates imbalances existing with your own hormones.

Women always ask me whether the hormones I recommend to my patients are really "natural." The question is really how do you define *natural*, a term that is very appealing to the public. But in the world of commerce, the term is often abused.

For me, *natural* means that the hormone is the exact chemical replica of what is produced in the body.

Premarin, the widely used estrogen prescription, contains estrogens extracted from the urine of pregnant horses. It may come from a natural source, but it is far from the same hormone you have in your body. It has different chemistry, and that difference is what makes it unnatural to me. It contains a dozen estrogen compounds, only one of which is a replica of what we have in the human body, while the others are foreign estrogens. Premarin is not an ideal solution for humans, though it might be fine for estrogen-deficient mares.

Many of the natural hormones that I and other antiaging physicians use, and which have gained considerable interest among women in recent years, are made from soybeans and wild yams. These plants contain unique compounds that are processed chemically and made into the identical hormones you yourself produce. However, when you eat soy or yams, your body cannot utilize the compounds as hormones.

Why soy and wild yams? I would be equally as enthusiastic if we could make exact replica hormones from quartz or backyard weeds. But nature has truly given us great gifts in these plants. They are the cheapest and most abundant commercial sources from which to readily extract compounds and turn them into exact replicas of our own hormones.

Today, we have access to many of these exact-replica hormones, either through prescription or over-the-counter. The body recognizes them as its very own hormones. It is this acceptance by the body that gives us a remarkable tool to replenish what is deficient or fluctuating in the system and restore healthful and youthful balances.

2

Hormones and Individuality

Individuality is the most important part of a hormone program. I never consider people according to how they fit into some artificial "normal" range. Some people have symptoms even though their blood tests are normal; others have no symptoms with levels considered too high or too low.

If you come to my office, you will see a very short doctor who stands five foot one. Shaquille O'Neal, the famous professional basketball player, towers more than seven feet tall. Science says that both of us are within the "normal" range for height, yet obviously I am very short and he is very tall. It doesn't matter that the medical system regards us both as being within a normal range. Neither one of us is actually normal.

Medical "report cards" have become a way of life. We are measured for height, weight, and "good" and "bad" cholesterol. If the numbers fall within normal, we are told to feel assured.

This heavy reliance on normal-range readings is nothing less than a tragic medical addiction. Many of these tests, including hormone tests, offer little more than quick and incomplete glances into the body's operation at certain frozen moments. If you take the test again at a later time, the biological and hormonal tides will have changed, and you may get altogether different readings.

When I treat a new patient I first obtain hormone level readings that serve as a baseline. I want to measure the levels not against any so-called normal range, but against how the patient is doing and how she feels at these hormone levels. It is against this background that I can plan hormonal strategy.

To illustrate my point let's create two make-believe patients, June and Rose, and a hypothetical hormone to give them. We'll call it hormone X and say that it brings fullness to the breasts, clears the mind, enhances mental focus, and prevents hot flashes.

11

June, the first patient, comes to my office and says her breasts are shrinking, her mind is foggy, and she has hot flashes. I test her and find that hormone X is within the normal range. Nevertheless, June has all the clinical signs of hormone X deficiency. The wide range of normal doesn't take into account that signs of deficiency or excess can still occur within normal parameters. I would recommend that June take extra natural hormone X to raise the level back to where she once was and I would expect to see her symptoms disappear. In order to function without symptoms, June might need to be in the 75th percentile of normal rather than in the 50th percentile.

Rose, our other hypothetical patient, has a much lower level of hormone X than June, but like June, she is also within the normal range. Rose, however, has no symptoms. She feels great. If I were to supplement her with hormone X, I might trigger all the undesirable side effects associated with an excess of the hormone.

For Rose, a relatively low level is fine. For June, a higher level—in comparison to Rose's—is a problem.

I relate the level of hormone X to symptoms or lack of symptoms. This tells me much more than relating it to an arbitrary low, normal, or high range. Moreover, some women need constant balancing in the face of wide hormonal fluctuations. Others, whose hormone levels are more stable, need less balancing.

The Art of Using Hormones

Using hormones is an individual art. This book will teach you to become an artist in perfecting and optimizing your intake.

When you don't take enough of a hormone, you don't get all the benefits. Only when you are close or in the optimum range, will you get the benefits. And if you go a little above your optimum zone, you will get a temporary side effect. The beauty of natural hormones is that your body speaks, and you learn to listen.

Your response to a hormone will be unique. You are different from your sister, your cousin, and your best friend: your immune system is different, your skin reacts differently, your gastrointestinal tract has particular strengths and weaknesses, and your vagina and breasts respond differently.

The specific dosage recommendations you will read later on in the book are based on the experiences of thousands of women. My patients all learn to adjust their own individual hormonal levels. Use these guidelines to find your own level. Learn what happens when you take too little or too much of a particular hormone. Learn how to deal with your own fluctuations. Learn how to balance yourself and stay in the optimum zone.

At every age of life, hormonal cycles operate differently. Our bodies are not like machines operating in a vacuum where one can precisely predict what the machine is going to do. Women with PMS don't have the same degree of PMS every month. The intensity of hot flashes varies from day to day.

Understand that your body has its own agenda. It reacts to external elements in your life and doesn't really inform you what it intends to do next. The level of hormone X you take may be fine for a few weeks, and then it may be too high or too low. The impact could be felt on your intellect, memory, mood, sleep, or energy.

You might think that there is something wrong with the hormone or that it isn't being absorbed well. But the problem may be that the dosage you need now is different. This book will help you learn how to read the messages your body delivers to you and how to adjust your dosage accordingly. It is not too complex.

Your body is like a moving, ever-changing needle. Your hormones are fluctuating, even as they diminish with age. This book will teach you to thread that needle, even as it keeps moving.

3

Before You Start—Tending to Your Stress and Insulin

STRESS, INSULIN, AND HEALTH

Chronic stress and faulty diets cause disease and accelerate aging. These are major health issues and should be addressed before attempting any new regimen.

Cortisol, the stress hormone, and insulin, the body's sugar-regulating hormone, play pivotal roles in your physiology. Studies have shown that many people living more than a hundred years tend to have low levels of cortisol and insulin, while many individuals who succumb to disease at a relatively young age have comparatively higher levels.

Chronic stress and high insulin interfere with normal hormone function. They also interfere with your ability to optimize the health and antiaging benefits of a natural hormone program.

Before you embark on a natural hormone program, I want to bring these issues to your attention, and offer some suggestions for dealing with them.

The Stress Connection

Stress, in our modern day society, is nothing less than an epidemic. One Gallup poll found that about a quarter of the American workforce suffers from an excess of stress and anxiety. One in five have stress-induced insomnia, and 15 percent of the population has an anxiety disorder.

One person among these statistics is my patient Sally, a superbusy entertainment industry executive. She arrived late for her afternoon appointment one day, visibly wearing the signs of a particularly busy and frustrating day.

14

I made some jokes and light talk in order to calm her down a little. Then we dealt with her hormonal issues. Before she left, I brought up the subject of stress.

I explained to her how all the good things she was doing with natural hormones were being nullified by her stress.

"The stress is going to make your skin more wrinkled, your brain more confused, and your memory less effective," I said to her. "It decreases the blood flow to your brain, undermines your immune system, and exhausts your antiaging hormones. It will make you sick and shorten your life."

"Well, I have all these people who depend on me and if I don't perform then it affects them," she said.

"It doesn't really matter who or what stresses you, and whether it is important or not important," I answered. "The effect on you is the same. The people around you all need you. Let them adjust to you. The worst thing you can do is get sicker quicker, lose your mind, and age faster."

I tend to give this sermon to all my patients who arrive in the office stressed. After all, they are there for antiaging treatment and advice. They may not expect to hear about stress, but they *need* to hear about it. Otherwise, they are really wasting their money.

Cortisol is the body's stress hormone, secreted by the adrenal glands. It is produced in response to stress. In the past, the hormone served us in times of danger, giving us bursts of extra strength and energy when we needed to fight or escape.

Today, we are generally not exposed to such life-threatening situations. But the same cortisol we would produce if a lion chased us is also produced by everyday stress that characterizes life in our modern age. There are many books and scientific articles describing the connection between stress and increased cortisol, disease and aging.

The bottom line is that stress is a killer.

Paul J. Rosch, M.D., president of the American Institute of Stress and clinical professor of medicine and psychiatry at New York Medical College, says there is no question that a chronic high tide of cortisol contributes to an acceleration of the aging process and a host of disorders.

In *Brain Longevity* (Warner Books), a book on maintaining peak mental performance, Dharma Singh Khalsa, M.D., emphasizes that chronic exposure of the brain to toxic levels of cortisol is a primary cause of brain degeneration, including Alzheimer's disease, during the aging process.

"When produced in excess, day after day—as a result of chronic, unrelenting stress—this hormone is so toxic to the brain that it kills and injures brain cells by the billions," he says.

If we could meditate every day, get a daily massage, eat food from our own garden, and live where the air and water were clean, we would be less affected by stress. Unfortunately, many of us can't manage a totally ideal lifestyle.

But we can all do some kind of stress damage control in our lives.

Stress has two components: the stressor (the cause) and the stressee (the person being stressed). Often you don't have control over the causes of stress in your life, but you have 100 percent control over the stressee—yourself.

Let me share with you a simple on-the-spot technique (see the box, "Breathe Your Stress Away") that works for me in the face of any stressful situation. It's a one- or two-step procedure, depending on how much time you have. If you don't have time for the first step, go directly to the second.

These simple exercises help eliminate a lot of unnecessary and prolonged stress. They help extinguish emotional fires at the moment of stress instead of letting them burn on until you go home to relax with a glass of wine or meditate.

I gave this technique to Sally, the entertainment executive, and it has helped her in her typically stressful work.

For some of my patients, I have noticed that even the process of aging itself can cause stress. As they start to see the signs of age they become anxious and worried. Brenda, a forty-five-year-old patient, is one of them.

Now and then she would complain to me about getting older. During one of her recent office visits, she was agonizing about it.

In my opinion, she is an absolutely gorgeous woman. But she believes that the people in her life see her today as a mere fading remnant of the stunning brunette she was twenty-five years ago.

"I wish I could give you a pill to knock this idea out of your head," I told her. "I see an utterly beautiful woman sitting in front of me. You turn the head of every man who sees you. Not one of them is wondering how much better you might have looked twenty years ago.

"You have the same soul you had years ago. Yet you are extinguishing it and the ageless inner beauty that enlivens and nourishes your outer beauty.

"If you keep this up you will indeed get old, sick, and dry up from the inside out. You are programming yourself to age because you think only about being older. Instead, you should see yourself for the magnificent woman you are today."

BREATHE YOUR STRESS AWAY

Step 1

Anytime you feel upset or agitated, just close your eyes and breathe deeply. Breathe in to the count of three. Then hold your breath for another count of three. And finally exhale to the count of three. Inhale. Hold. Exhale. Your breathing will become slower, deeper, more regular.

If you can do this deep breathing technique for a few times you will actually be putting control back into your brain.

If you can do it for five minutes or longer, that's even better. It becomes like a meditation. Just observe your breathing as you breathe in and out. Don't try to alter it. The rhythm may speed up or slow down. It may get deeper or more shallow. It may even seem to stop for a time.

You will find that at times your attention drifts away from your breath and goes to a thought in your mind, a sensation in your body, or a sound in the environment. Whenever you notice that you are not observing the breath, gently and innocently bring your attention back to your breathing.

When you finish, wait about a minute before you slowly open your eyes.

If you can't do the deep breathing for a few minutes, then do it at least for a few times and go directly to step 2.

Step 2

Take a deep breath. While you inhale, envision yourself at your funeral looking very old in the casket, much older than all the friends and family members of the same age who are in attendance. When you exhale, envision people saying that it was a good thing you died because you looked so old and your brain was no longer functional.

The funeral scenario works great for me. When I finish exhaling I automatically become stronger in my resolve not to allow the particular stressful situation to push me closer to my grave where people will see me die young yet looking like an old man with no brain function.

And, I added with a laugh, "If you don't think you are beautiful, what does that make me?"

I told Brenda that from my individual perspective as a male I see women continuing to be beautiful no matter what their age.

"My wife is more beautiful to me now than she was thirty years ago," I said. "She may pack a few more pounds on her hips and have more lines on her face, but that doesn't matter. She has other things I love about her now that she didn't have then."

When I finished talking, I think Brenda felt better. She thanked me. In subsequent visits, she said she has been working on aging gracefully.

We all have to learn to accept ourselves as we are and not punish ourselves for being older. If we don't, we just create stress. And stress, for sure, will age us even more. Using natural hormones helps improve and delay the aging process, and preserve youthfulness, but any kind of stress will cancel out such benefits.

Obviously, stress is a very complex issue, and I don't mean to imply that one conversation with your doctor or a simple breathing technique will protect you from it. Regular meditation, prayer, yoga, massage, small breaks from the daily routine, and exercise all have been shown to improve the body's ability to cope with stress. Stress is a major medical and antiaging issue. Do not shrug it off. Find something that works for you.

Among the hormones covered in this book, melatonin, DHEA, pregnenolone, and human growth hormone are particularly beneficial for chronic stress. I discuss these hormones in part four.

I also recommend the following supplements to my patients for additional stress protection. They are available in health food stores.

The Insulin Connection

Insulin and low blood sugar problems are often the cause of fatigue, irritability, depression, mood swings, poor memory and confusion, dizziness, low sex drive, and craving for sweets. These irregularities can be the underlying reasons why many women who take hormones do not have good results.

Blood sugar (also called glucose) serves as the fuel—just like the gasoline that runs your car—for the cells that generate mental and physical activity. Without an adequate and steady supply of fuel, you experience muscle weakness and a wide array of physiological problems.

A genetic weakness or an excess intake of grains and highly processed foods, particularly carbohydrates and sweets, can cause lots of trouble. These foods are broken down into sugar and cause roller-coaster reactions in the body.

The pancreas secretes the hormone insulin to control the sugar level in the blood. Insulin moves the sugar into the cells for use in energy production. When the body is flooded with sugar, the pancreas responds with a high level of insulin. This drives the blood sugar level lower. As a result, your energy can plummet immediately after a meal to a state of fatigue. Your mood can swing

STRESS-BUSTING SUPPLEMENTS

Phosphatidylserine

This naturally occurring substance is a major component of cell membranes and is most concentrated in the brain. Among the conclusions reached in more than sixty-five human studies, phosphatidylserine helps revitalize the aging brain and protect the brain from stress. Take 300 milligrams daily with meals. I recommend 100 milligrams with breakfast and 200 milligrams with dinner.

Adrenal Support Formula

Choose a supplement containing adrenal tissue extracts, pantothenic acid, and B complex. Follow label instructions.

Magnesium Glycinate

Magnesium is a great natural relaxant. Most people are, in fact, deficient in this important mineral. Stress burns up the body's magnesium stores. Research shows that your body actually responds worse to stress if you are deficient in magnesium. Supplementation helps combat PMS symptoms. Start with 250 milligrams a day and increase your dosage to 250 milligrams up to three times a day, or as tolerated. If you take too much you will develop drowsiness or frequent bowel movements. Take with meals.

Adaptogens Such as Ginseng

Follow label instructions. Panax or American ginseng was traditionally consumed by American Indians as a general tonic and restorative, and to help the mind. Today, American ginseng is known for its adaptogenic properties—its ability to bring balance to a distressed system. Panax is considered by the Chinese as the most sacred of all herbs. Unlike Siberian or Korean ginseng, which have more stimulating effects (yang), American ginseng is more sedative and relaxing (yin energy) in its action.

Kava

This South Pacific herb promotes relaxation without affecting mental sharpness. I recommend the herb in an oral spray form that can be used throughout the day before or after stressful events.

from euphoria to irritability and depression. These blood sugar fluctuations often go by the name of hypoglycemia.

Over time the constant overproduction of insulin creates a condition called hyperinsulinemia and can lead to serious metabolic disturbances throughout the body, including insulin resistance and diabetes. The elevated insulin stimulates the release of substances appropriately named AGES—advanced glycosated end products. These sugar molecules enter into cells and interfere with cellular operations, including the ability of the cells to receive and process the chemical information delivered by insulin and other hormones.

Elevated insulin causes the body to have great difficulty breaking down fat. Weight gain results. Other consequences include increased blood pressure and the promotion of free radical activity, biochemical reactions in the body that accelerate aging and the development of disease.

Individuals who suspect an insulin problem should consult with a physician and undergo a simple insulin level test. After not eating overnight, and abstaining from breakfast, have a blood sample drawn. Ideally, you want an insulin level in the range of 5, and below 10 mcu/ml. Above 10 means potential problems, over 15 is considered hyperinsulinemia. Higher than 30 is overt diabetes. In my experience with my patients, balancing insulin definitely improves hormonal treatment.

From a practical standpoint, there are some concrete steps you can take to prevent the high tide of insulin in your body.

The following table—called a glycemic index—details a range of commonly eaten foods that break down into sugar the fastest and cause the biggest rush of insulin in the body. Of course, sweets are among them. But you will also be surprised to see the names of foods here that are otherwise considered good and wholesome. The idea is to minimize such foods as much as possible, particularly if you do have a blood sugar problem.

The glycemic index was developed in 1981 by David Jenkins, a University of Toronto nutritionist, and has become widely recognized among nutritionally oriented physicians. The index assigns numerical values to different carbohydrates that indicate how fast they are broken down and become glucose in the body. The higher the number the faster the food turns to glucose and raises your blood sugar level. All foods are rated in comparison to glucose itself, which has a 100 value.

Keep in mind that the impact foods have on blood sugar is influenced also by its fat and fiber content (they slow the process down), ripeness, cooking time, time of day, blood insulin level, and recent activity. You are probably not going to keep a glycemic account every time you sit down to eat, however familiarizing yourself with this concept can help you control your blood sugar. This is not a diet book, but unless you eliminate high glycemic foods in the presence of an insulin problem you may not have good results from natural hormones.

In the table, I also include a sampling of some of the low glycemic index foods for comparison, that is, foods that break down more slowly.

THE GLYCEMIC INDEX

puffed rice	90	oatmeal	53
white rice	88	apples	52
Rice Krispies	82	whole rye	50
waffle	76	ice cream	50
white bread	72	pumpernickel	49
whole wheat	72	orange	43
bagel	72	baked beans	43
oatmeal (instant)	66	milk	34
rye	64	lima beans	32
raisins	64	split peas	32
bananas	62	black beans	30
bran muffin	60	banana (unripe)	30
brown rice	59	kidney beans	27
apple juice	58	soybeans	18
sweet corn	55		

For patients who have problems controlling their sweet tooth, I often recommend a combination of specific nutritional supplements to help bring sugar cravings under control and thus help reduce the insulin level.

SUGAR-CRAVING BUSTERS

- **Chromium picolinate.** Take 200 micrograms, three times daily a half hour before meals.
- **Alpha lipoic acid.** Take 100 to 250 milligrams, three times daily a half hour before meals.
- **Vanadyl sulfate.** Take 10 milligrams, three times daily a half hour before meals.
- **Magnesium glycinate.** Take 250 milligrams up to three times a day (or as tolerated) with meals.
- **Gymnema sylvestre.** Take a standardized extract of this Ayurvedic herb twice a day.

Every patient who has taken these few supplements, eliminated high glycemic foods, and introduced more protein and healthy fats into their diet has been able to reduce insulin-related problems and increase the benefits of a natural hormone program.

4

Making Your Physician a Natural Hormone Partner

Today's managed care medical environment has made it tougher on a physician's professional life. Besides the stress, pressure, and responsibility involved, doctors face so many hazards on the job that they should probably begin wearing hard hats to work. I don't know a single group of professionals that is more harassed, regulated, and unappreciated.

Unless you see an antiaging or preventive medicine specialist, it is unlikely that your doctor will have the knowledge, ability, or time to help you fine-tune your hormones. We live in an age of crisis medicine. *Most people go to their doctors with problems and not with the intent to prevent problems.*

This is a flawed system, and a flawed emphasis. You only have to look at a few statistics to realize how badly flawed. I'll share three statistics with you here:

- The 1996 University of San Francisco study that found about ninety-nine million Americans suffer from some form of chronic ailment. That's 40 percent of the population!
- Up to two million Americans are hospitalized, and about 100,000 die each year, from the side effects of prescription drugs.
- Ninety-nine percent of the government's "health sector budget" is used to treat illness after it occurs. One percent is allocated for prevention, even though the vast majority of chronic illnesses are preventable. Health care reform bills basically deal with who will pay for whose disease and how to streamline disease-care financing and delivery. There's no talk of improving health.

Even against this dismal background, if your physician goes off the beaten path of primarily pharmaceutical and surgical choices, the insurance establishment may not pay for it. And the medical establishment doesn't really like it.

A physician's freedom to choose different techniques or remedies that are not "officially sanctioned" is often quite limited. If he or she chooses "alternatives," there may be a job risk involved, no matter how effective the treatment is and how much it helps patients.

Fortunately, this situation is improving, thanks to a large and growing patient demand for safer and more effective options. In recent years we have seen a huge influx of patients resorting to "alternative" practitioners along with a parallel integration of "alternative" methods by many conventional doctors.

Despite the changing climate, don't be surprised if your interest in natural hormones falls on deaf ears. Most physicians aren't familiar with natural hormones. They aren't familiar with how natural hormones can help many typical female problems or address aging concerns.

Try to work with your doctor. Show him or her this book. Explain that it gives step-by-step details about what to do and how to monitor progress. Hopefully your physician will at least write the prescriptions you need and monitor you with standard medical tests.

Natural hormones are legal to prescribe and use, and increasing numbers of doctors are recommending them because of their safety and effectiveness. They offer a powerful alternative to "conventional" pharmaceutical hormonal prescriptions that may cause imbalances and side effects.

There are hundreds of compounding pharmacies around the country that can fill natural hormone prescriptions for you. You will need prescriptions for estrogen, progesterone, as well as for testosterone and human growth hormones, if you choose to use them.

Compounding pharmacists mix, assemble and package prescriptions to meet the individualized needs of patients. The local pharmacist you may be more familiar with is likely to dispense the manufactured form of a particular medication. Both types of pharmacists are fully licensed.

The two particular compounding pharmacies I use fill natural hormone prescriptions written by thousands of other doctors all over the country. Very knowledgeable professionals staff the pharmacies and can provide your doctor with any needed information.

If your doctor is reluctant to become actively involved in a natural hormone program with you, just ask for a few months' time to see how you fare.

The results may win him or her over. In this book, I have tried to cover many contingencies and situations encountered by a wide variety of women who take natural hormones. The information here can also guide your physician. It is based on years of clinical experience with thousands of patients.

If your doctor won't write a prescription or authorize the medical tests, please be understanding. In such a case, you may prefer to seek out a physician near you who prescribes natural hormones. Compounding pharmacies can give you names and numbers of practitioners in your area. You can also find a practitioner through the American Academy of Anti-Aging Medicine. Refer to Appendix A on how to contact these resources.

The physician you contact may have limited experience in balancing hormones and may only write a prescription and provide the requested tests for you. Another physician may have more knowledge of female hormones and be able to help you fine-tune your hormones. In either case, the guidelines in this book cover most contingencies and should enable you to achieve optimum balance on your own.

Regarding insurance, your health plan may or may not cover the tests. Some plans have contracts with compounding pharmacies. If your plan does not cover natural hormones, I would strongly urge you to complain and point out the major problems associated with patented, chemicalized hormonal substitutes. If enough people complain, the companies will listen. If your plan won't cover your tests, than find an accredited medical laboratory and have the tests done yourself. I describe the tests throughout the book.

I believe that physicians everywhere can embrace the safe and effective program in this book. Natural hormones can benefit both practitioner and patients.

PART TWO

How to Control Estrogen—Instead of Being Controlled

5

ABCs of Estrogen

Estrogen at a Glance

The Role of Estrogen—the Essence of Femininity

Estrogen, as *Time* magazine said in a 1995 cover article, is "powerful stuff." It is the hormone that shapes the uniqueness of your mind, emotions, and body. It is estrogen that ignites the physical transformation from childhood to womanhood. During the menstrual cycle it generates the proper womb environment for implantation and nourishment of the early embryo.

Estrogen makes you feel sensual. It brings glow to the skin, moisture to the eyes, fullness to the breasts, and clarity to the mind. It keeps the vagina lubricated. It uplifts and stabilizes your mood. It influences your brain and your bones, and protects you against cardiovascular disease.

There are, in fact, more than three hundred tissue systems throughout the body where estrogen has a major impact.

The sexuality associated with estrogen should not be misunderstood. It is not the hormone of orgasmic power and passion. It relates more to the feeling of female pride, vitality, and sensuality. It is this essence of feminine

27

energy and sensuality that differentiates a woman from the girl she used to be. And it is this same essence that ebbs with the years when the level of estrogen declines in the adult woman. With the increasing loss of estrogen, it seems that many women start giving up on their youthfulness and "woman-ness." In many ways, menopause is a reversal of the adolescent transformation.

I am convinced that if a woman maintains a certain level of estrogen she can delay and somewhat arrest the changes associated with hormonal decline and deficiency. Estrogen replacement can restore much of her lost female uniqueness.

Estrogen is primarily formed in the ovaries and is a combination of three compounds: estrone (E1), estradiol (E2), and estriol (E3). Because of this unique three-in-one structure, estrogen is sometimes described in plural terms as "estrogens."

Currently, estrogen is "under attack" as a major risk factor in the epidemic of breast cancer. I find this ludicrous. Estrogen is the hormone that distinguishes women's unique gender.

After two million years of human evolution, could the female hormone suddenly have turned into a serial killer? Would nature suddenly decide to create a one-gender species? Of course not. Incriminating estrogen is as logical as saying that your liver is the cause of liver cancer.

Understanding Estrogen Fluctuations

For much of your life, estrogen fluctuates up and down. This occurs within the monthly cycle and also within the general framework of a lifetime. The degree and pattern of fluctuations are totally unique to you. So, too, are the ways your body reacts to the episodes of deficiencies and excesses created by the fluctuations.

Deficiency-related responses are much more common than responses resulting from excess. Following are symptoms of both deficiency and excess, along with typical comments from my patients.

Common Signs of Estrogen Deficiency
- Mental fogginess. "I've lost my mind."
- Forgetfulness. "I can't remember the birthdays of my grandchildren anymore."
- Depression. "It's like I'm living in a dark tunnel."
- Minor anxiety. "I can't seem to control my worries."

- Mood change. "Sometimes I wonder how I'm going to feel tomorrow."
- Difficulty falling asleep. "My mind is racing and I can't stop it."
- Hot flashes. "This wave of heat spreads through my body."
- Night sweats. "I wake up soaking wet."
- Temperature swings. "I feel like a broken air conditioner."
- Day-long fatigue. "I can't keep my head up."
- Reduced stamina. "I can't push it like I used to."
- Decreased sense of sexuality and sensuality. "I have lost all pride in my body."
- Lessened self-image and attention to appearance. "I could care less how I look."
- Dry eyes, skin, and vagina. "My body is like a dry summer."
- Loss of skin radiance. "I've lost my skin glow."
- Sense of normalcy only during second week of cycle: "I am myself only one week out of the month."
- Sagging breasts and loss of fullness. "These aren't the breasts I used to have."
- Pain with sexual activity. "I'm not lubricating as well."
- Weight gain, with increasing lack of concern about it. "I'm like a balloon that can't pop."
- Increased back and joint pain. "My body is stiff and hurts."
- Episodes of rapid heartbeat, with or without anxiety. "Out of nowhere my chest feels strained and I get palpitations."
- Headaches and migraines. "I seem to be controlled by pain that I never knew before."
- Gastrointestinal discomfort. "I feel bloated."

Some of the above reactions occur nearly simultaneously whenever the level of estrogen falls. Most notable are hot flashes, inability to sleep, mental fogginess, and emotional instability. The surprising news is that the symptoms improve very quickly as well, often within a half hour to an hour and a half after giving the body what it's missing: estrogen.

Common Signs of Excess Estrogen
- Breast tenderness or pain, occurring mainly in the central area, including the nipple: "My breasts are too painful even to touch."
- Increase of breast size. "My breasts are swollen."
- Water retention (as noticed in swollen fingers and legs). "I can't put on my rings."

- Impatient, snappy behavior, but with a clear mind. "People tell me I'm too bossy."
- Pelvic cramps, with or without uterine bleeding. "I'm back to cramps again like when I was younger."
- Nausea (less frequently). "I start to feel like I did when I was pregnant."

A woman with a high level of estrogen who is short-tempered and impatient tends to be in full control of her mind. Her thinking is crisp and clear. By comparison, an impatient woman with low estrogen often lacks the same mental sharpness and may experience mental fogginess.

I often tell women that when their estrogen is low, they are more apt to receive sympathy and forgiveness. When it is high, they seem to have greater potential to irritate others and not be forgiven.

There is a group of women, perhaps 5 percent, who naturally produce a high level of estrogen or who take a very large dosage of estrogen replacement without showing any sign of excess.

In addition to monthly cyclicity and age-related fluctuations, the following can cause symptoms related to an increase in estrogen:

- use of birth control pills
- hormonal replacement with a higher level of estrogen than needed
- fertility injections
- the presence of benign ovarian cysts.

Unlike low estrogen, which can produce more immediate effects, the signs of elevated estrogen develop more slowly, over three to five days.

If you take too much estrogen, or if your natural level is too high, or if the estrogen is not properly balanced with adequate progesterone, the lining of the uterus—the endometrium—will thicken. In response, the uterus will contract, inducing uterine bleeding and a sensation of pain or cramping in the lower pelvic area.

Learning to balance your estrogen level will help you avoid uterine bleeding and the potential for irritability.

How Do Your Fluctuations Affect You?

The first step to mastering, balancing, and optimizing your hormones is to understand how estrogen affects you. To do that, think about the estrogen-related changes in your life. Make a note of any of the responses you have had to estrogen highs and lows over the years.

Try to remember, for instance, the changes or symptoms you experienced as you went from a girl to a woman, the changes or symptoms related to your period, and the changes and symptoms related to getting older.

Keep an ongoing record. A personal hormonal history can be very useful to both you and your personal physician. Your reactions will provide important clues and the basis for comparison as you adjust and master your hormonal levels. Your own hormonal history will help you recognize if you are taking too much estrogen or too little.

As I said earlier, I have difficulty with the concept of "normal range." The result of a hormonal blood test may place you in a normal range. But what is normal for one woman may be high, or low, for another. The production of estrogen, as well as its fluctuations, its rate of decline, and its response to changes, are all very individual. Some women maintain higher levels for a longer period of time. In some women, the fluctuations and decline take a heavy toll on their physical, mental, and emotional well-being. In other women, the changes are felt only minimally.

The more familiar you become with your personal estrogen story, the more readily you will learn how to fine-tune your hormonal replacement program. And the more in touch you are with the uniqueness of your body, the more you can assist your physician to aid you in the process.

If you start a natural estrogen replacement program early, you will be better able to avoid the discomforts of fluctuations and the symptoms of the age-related estrogen decline. You will also be better able to preserve and enhance all the wonderful estrogen influences that make you so unique. To help you formulate your estrogen history, consider your reactions in relation to the fluctuations caused by the following situations or practices. Not every point presented here will pertain to you.

1. The Monthly Cycle

The monthly cycle—and how you feel throughout your cycle—is a good starting point for learning to self-adjust your hormonal level and create balance in your body.

First, the basics: the normal twenty-eight day cycle starts with the initial heavy flow of menstruation, day one. During a woman's period the estrogen level is very low. It starts to increase after menstruation and rises to its monthly peak on the day of ovulation, usually day fourteen. After ovulation there is a slow decline, followed by a slight peaking again around day twenty-one (a week after ovulation). At this point, if conception has not occurred, the production of estrogen again falls. The drop continues and reaches the cyclic bottom again on day one.

During the cycle there are wide fluctuations in the quantity of estrogen the body produces. There are also wide differences in the quantity of estrogen that different women produce.

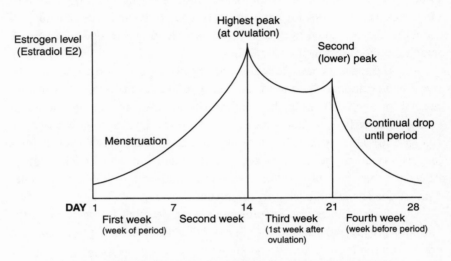

ESTROGEN PRODUCTION DURING THE MONTHLY CYCLE

How do you feel during your monthly fluctuations? If you feel best from day seven to day fourteen, that means your body likes a high level of estrogen. If you feel good only during this period, you are very probably estrogen deficient and will benefit from an estrogen replacement program.

How do you feel a few days before and during the period? This is when your estrogen level falls sharply—down to its monthly low. Women who usually suffer from deficiency of estrogen will have specific symptoms at this time.

How do you feel from the day of ovulation to the onset of heavy flow? This is when your body produces progesterone. Some women develop specific symptoms during this time of the month. The symptoms can change at different ages. This indicates a hormonal imbalance that I will discuss in the section on progesterone.

2. Changes during Puberty

Recall the transformations that occurred during your passage into womanhood—the mental, emotional, and interpersonal changes, and the appreciation of your body. These aspects of your persona can reverse as estrogen declines.

3. Pregnancy

Pregnancy is a time when the body dramatically steps up its production of estrogen. Can you recall how you felt during the second trimester? That will give you another clue to your estrogen individuality.

Did you feel better than before you became pregnant? If so, that indicates you were probably low in estrogen to begin with.

Did you feel worse than before you became pregnant? If so, you probably have little tolerance for an excess of estrogen. It is likely that you had a relatively higher level in your menstrual cycle.

Don't regard the first trimester as a yardstick. Many women do not feel well at all, regardless of their estrogen levels.

4. Women on the Birth Control Pill

The pill contains chemicalized estrogen that suppresses your own natural production.

Did you develop signs of deficiency after starting the pill? If so, that means you didn't get enough estrogen in the pill to compensate for the loss of your own naturally occurring estrogen. Many young women today are prescribed oral contraceptives with very low estrogen. This often causes deficiency symptoms. Such women need a stronger pill because they naturally produce a higher level of estrogen.

Did you feel miserable, gain weight, or experience an increase in breast size? That's an indication you probably had a low to average level of estrogen before starting the pill and didn't tolerate the additional estrogen in the pill.

Did you feel better after starting the pill? That means you probably were relatively low in estrogen to begin with but responded positively to a higher level.

Keep a record of the kind of pill you received—the brand, the types of hormone drugs it contained, and the dose. Your reaction to the estrogen in the pill will be very useful for a medical caregiver treating you years from now. It will give clues as to how your body responds to increased or decreased amounts of estrogen.

5. Women between Twenty-five and Forty-five

During this time there is a gradual, but significant, decline of estrogen. The decline is very individual. According to research, the average falloff from prior peak production is about one-third. There is also a parallel reduction in fertility.

Again, keep track of estrogen-related changes during this time. If you have passed this stage, do you recall any symptoms?

6. Perimenopause and Early Menopause

At this point in life, many women experience a hormonal roller coaster. Estrogen decline accelerates, not as a straight downward plunge, but more like a downhill alpine ski run, full of bumps and dips, some big, some small. You may go from significant overproduction to underproduction, sometimes within a single day. The fluctuations create a range of reactions that will vary in intensity and frequency.

Initially, reactions are more significant. Over time, they tend to decrease in intensity and frequency.

Some women may undergo maximum drops in their hormonal level yet hardly experience any symptoms at all. Others may have minimum drops and develop a broadside of symptoms at one time. Others may experience a sequence of symptoms, while others only one symptom.

7. Over Sixty

Menopause-related changes generally diminish. There is little fluctuation in estrogen as the remaining hormone level slowly sinks further.

8. Chemical or Surgical Menopause

Chemical menopause, when the ovaries stop working because of the damaging effect of chemotherapy, or surgical menopause, when the ovaries are removed, also cause sudden changes. I will talk about these situations in chapter 8.

Estrogen and the Shape of Your Body

A woman's shape and breast size during her younger years serve as a superb yardstick of estrogen production. These details suggest how much of the hormone she may need in a replacement program.

For this purpose, we use three categories of body types. Types one and two experience *very different* physiological responses to high or low estrogen.

Estrogen Type One: Short, Voluptuous, and Full-Breasted

This woman produces more estrogen. She functions on a relatively higher level. The abundance of estrogen creates larger breasts, earlier bone closure, and smaller stature.

She does not tolerate further increases in estrogen. This is why she feels uncomfortable on a strong birth control pill or during the second trimester of pregnancy. However, a birth control pill of low potency might create some signs of deficiency.

This woman needs a relatively higher level of estrogen replacement during menopause.

Estrogen Type Two: Taller, Thinner, and Relatively Small-Breasted

Here, the woman operates on much less estrogen and usually develops her period later. She has grown taller because of less estrogen in the system to promote the calcification of bone tissue. Smaller breast size is a sign of relatively lower estrogen.

Many of these women have totally adapted to low estrogen. They may not feel the cyclic drop of estrogen as intensely as shorter, full-breasted females do. Some may experience chronic and subtle signs of estrogen deficiency that become more pronounced just before and during their period.

A type two woman generally feels wonderful during pregnancy or when taking the birth control pill. Both situations elevate the overall estrogen level.

During menopause, a relatively lower level of estrogen is needed.

Estrogen Type Three: "In-betweeners"

Here we find the largest number of women. They produce an average amount of estrogen, with some tending toward the high end and others toward the low end.

PHYSIOLOGICAL NEEDS VS. DOSING TRENDS

The current prescribing trend is to give women lower and lower doses of estrogen. This may be fine for the person who requires a small amount of estrogen replacement. But it won't resolve the needs for someone who needs much more. It will still perpetuate their deficiency and deprivation.

There are major differences in the physiological needs for estrogen among women. Your individuality cannot be addressed by a low-dose, fixed-dose standard.

The estrogen replacement needs of a tall, thin, flat-chested woman are totally different from those of a shorter, full-breasted female. Their reactions are also different.

The Modern Dilemma of Estrogen "Dominance"

The body produces three estrogen compounds. Each has different tasks to perform. Two of them—estrone (E1) and estradiol (E2)—are the so-called aggressive types of estrogen. At high levels, they are thought to be associated with increased risk of breast and uterine cancer, and as a result they have been made scapegoats for the proliferation of breast cancer (see chapter 23 for more on this subject).

The two compounds tend to convert back and forth into each other. For that reason, the standard blood test for estrogen is based on the estradiol value only.

We regard estrone and estradiol as the most influential estrogens in creating the qualities of femininity, the qualities that turn a girl into a woman and affect and protect the mind, the bones, and the cardiovascular system. Estradiol prevents loss of old bone tissue. Estrone is thought to perhaps promote new bone tissue.

Estriol (E3), the third major type of estrogen, is the more "benign" compound. It contributes to healthy and youthful skin, keeps the vagina lubricated, prevents hot flashes and night sweats, and probably has a major anticancer role. It exerts a protective and counterbalancing effect against estradiol and estrone, its more powerful sister compounds. In some women I find that the only way to improve mental clarity is to increase the replacement level of estriol. Some women respond better to estriol in the gel form, while others do better with either sublingual drops or capsules. Estriol does not appear to benefit the bones or cardiovascular system.

During pregnancy there is a dramatic rise in the levels of estrogen compounds. Most significant of all is the rise in estriol. This reproductive mode also generates extra progesterone, which acts as a further protector against the "aggressive" estrogens (estradiol and estrone). Indeed, the overall balance of elevated hormones during pregnancy offers considerable protection for the female body. Research amply shows that the more full-term pregnancies a woman has in her life, the lower her risk of developing breast and ovarian cancer, endometriosis, cysts, and fibroids. In a way these conditions can be viewed as modern female diseases, a result of women choosing birth control and fewer pregnancies over the historical pattern of multiple childbirth.

Seen from a historical perspective, the "normal" monthly menstruation cycles and fewer pregnancies of modern women are basically abnormal. The modern cycles and reduced pregnancies, along with other factors, contribute to an accumulation of "aggressive" estrogens in the body. We call this situation estrogen "dominance." Here's how it develops:

1. Women produce "aggressive" estrogen every day of the month.
2. They do not produce enough protective estriol.
3. Progesterone, which protects the body and balances estrogen, is produced only during the two weeks of the month following ovulation.
4. The level of progesterone declines significantly after a woman reaches thirty-five.
5. During perimenopause, progesterone is usually gone from the body.
6. The birth control pill that liberates women from the risk of pregnancy could raise the level of aggressive estrogen in their bodies. The pill contains only strong, chemicalized estrogens along with chemicalized progestin, which has no resemblance to your natural progesterone. Thus, the pill gives you aggressive estrogen without estriol or progesterone protection.
7. Unlike any time before in history, we are exposed today to huge amounts of "xenoestrogens"—foreign estrogens originating outside the body. Pesticides and chemical compounds found in plastics, detergents, personal care products, canned food, and even contraceptive creams contain these xenoestrogens. Dioxin is one such chemical, a dangerous compound found throughout the environment and in alarming levels in our food supply. These chemicals behave like an aggressive estrogen and further throw hormonal levels off balance. They often begin creating problems in young girls. The body reacts to such estrogens by triggering the sexual transformation well before the thirteen or fourteen years that was the natural, evolutionary norm. Today, females come into menses at an earlier age than ever, some as young as nine.

Problems most likely influenced by estrogen dominance include the rise of breast, ovarian, and uterine cancer, as well as the high incidence of endometriosis, fibroids, and adenomyosis, a benign inward growth of the lining of the uterus.

From 1972 to 1976, I practiced in Israel, in an area where most women followed a traditional pattern of multiple pregnancies. My patients included Palestinians as well as North African and religious Jewish women. I rarely saw any of the conditions that we commonly see today in gynecological practice. They didn't have cancer, menstrual cramps, abnormal bleeding, PMS, migraines, fibroids, adenomyosis, or endometriosis. Their main complaint was that after so many pregnancies, they often had varicose veins and a prolapse of the uterus.

In our society, only a small percentage of women choose to reproduce at this rate—every eighteen months or two years, and raise ten to seventeen children. Obviously, I am not advocating this as a solution to the dilemma of estrogen dominance.

A practical solution is the use of natural hormones. They can restore balance. They can prevent the buildup of "aggressive" estrogens and the threat of estrogen. As you read along, your options will become very clear.

A Little Necessary Endocrinology

I don't want to burden you with the complexities of endocrinology, the study of hormonal secretions. However, I must introduce you to something called the "sex hormone–binding globulin." This unheralded protein can make a big difference in your understanding and control of your hormones. So take a deep breath and indulge me in this little necessary foray into endocrinology.

The inner intelligence of your body doesn't want hormones running wild or falling below a certain level. It wants normalcy, hormonal law and order. To achieve this, your body utilizes a team of specialized proteins produced by the liver.

These proteins chaperone individual hormone molecules through the blood. Should the hormones reach too high a level, the protein binds and inactivates them—sort of like a handcuffing effect. The protein not only transports but also regulates and assists in the access process at target cell sites.

Estrogen's chaperone is the sex hormone-binding globulin (SHBG). When your estrogen level goes too high, an alarm goes off in the liver, the body's master chemical factory. It pumps out extra SHBG. In reaction to a high tide of estrogen, your liver can produce up to three times the normal amount of SHBG.

The problem is that this special protein doesn't just bind up some of the excess estrogen. It also binds—and inactivates—some of the other important hormones, such as thyroid hormone, human growth hormone, and testosterone.

For example let's say your body normally has 10 milligrams of thyroid hormone in circulation: 5 milligrams are free, available to act on cells throughout the body, and 5 are bound up by SHBG. Now, your liver steps up production of SHBG in order to control your excess estrogen. While curbing the estrogen, it also curbs thyroid hormone. So now 8 milligrams of thyroid hormone are bound up, leaving the body only 2 in use.

The effect on you is not immediate. It takes about six weeks before you usually start to experience fallout from the lowered hormonal activity. The consequences are highly variable. Quantities of your important antiaging hormones have now been taken out of commission. In essence, the available amount of these hormones falls to levels you might have when you are many years older. The body becomes less "alive." Perhaps the skin becomes less radiant, the vagina drier. Lowered thyroid, for instance, can cause weight gain, fatigue, coldness, and dry skin. These are all signs of thyroid deficiency. Elevated SHBG can cause such multiple effects.

Why are these endocrine details important? Because SHBG may be the reason—and the answer—that you don't feel well when you start estrogen replacement. This may be the key to helping you achieve overall hormonal balance.

When you take estrogen orally or rub it into the skin, the body doesn't know that it comes from the outside. Your internal radar picks up the added estrogen, thinks it is produced from within, and responds by mobilizing more sex hormone–binding globulin. Maybe in fifty thousand years our body will be smart enough to discriminate. But you can't wait that long.

The surge of SHBG is especially dramatic after you take estrogen by mouth. Please remember this: oral estrogen, primarily in the form of pills, proceeds from your mouth down into the digestive tract. From there it is carried, as a high tide of estrogen, directly to the liver. The liver now thinks there is way too much estrogen in your system. The alarm goes off. Out swarm the sex hormone–binding globulins like a SWAT team.

Thus, if you take estrogen in this way, you don't receive the full benefit of the dosage. You actually need more, because the higher SHBG has bound up more of the circulating estrogen in your body, whether you produced it in your ovaries or took it orally. In other words, the SHBG cancels out more of the estrogen along with other hormones.

This does not happen, or happens to a much, much smaller degree when you take estrogen in other forms, such as topical gel or patch.

When the estrogen level plunges, as in menopause or during breast-feeding, SHBG activity goes down. Your body understands the emotional and physical duress associated with exceptionally low estrogen. It now tries to compensate by raising the levels of other hormones. Going back to our previous example, we find that instead of binding 5 milligrams of thyroid or other hormones, the body unlocks more of these hormones for use in the body. It may bind only 2 milligrams of each. Thus, as a woman ages, and her estrogen levels naturally decrease, the grip of SHBG loosens.

This issue will enter into your consideration of *how* to take natural estrogen in order to balance your hormones. In addition, the level of SHBG in your body can be monitored by a blood test and used by your physician as a clue to hormonal status.

The interplay between SHBG and hormones can be quite complex. Technically, each hormone has its own specific sex hormone–binding globulin, but they all are affected directly or indirectly by the estrogen level and how estrogen is administered.

Thank you for sitting through this little lesson in endocrinology. Just remember the following:

- SHBG binds up more hormones when estrogen rises.
- SHBG releases more hormones when estrogen goes down.

6

Problems with Conventional Estrogen Replacement (ERT)

Estrogen replacement therapy (ERT) is widely prescribed when signs of significant deficiency develop, such as at complete menopause, or when the ovaries are removed surgically or cease to function due to chemotherapy.

Pharmaceutical companies today make most of the estrogen products available to women. I have nothing against pharmaceutical companies—they make major contributions to the comfort and health of women in our society—but I can't for the life of me understand their approach to hormonal replacement.

Hormones are fundamental biological substances in the function of our bodies. They have been part of our physiology ever since human life first stirred on this planet. When you have such exquisite substances that have worked for so long, and you have the ability to duplicate them exactly, why create substitutes? And why create substitutes based on estrogen extracted from the urine of a horse, the FDA-approved estrogen standard?

Obviously, when pharmaceutical companies put a lot of time and money into research, development, and marketing, they seek a good return for their investment. So they research and create a synthetic substitute. They produce it under the protection of a patent because they don't want other companies to copy what they have developed at great expense.

I strongly believe that pharmaceutical companies could make the same profits, and probably more, if they would just give to women the precise ingredients that their bodies need instead of unnatural substitutes. Pharmaceutical companies could have countless happy female customers who would use much more of their products. And as an important bonus, there would be a huge reduction in side effects and medical complications.

Statistics indicate that 50 percent of patients do not use the hormonal prescriptions their doctors write for them. In addition, of those who do fill their prescriptions, less than 40 percent continue to take the hormonal medications beyond one year. This represents an immense population seeking other options.

Unfortunately, the designers of hormonal replacement do not get the message. They think the lack of compliance is due to the difficulty of taking two different hormones (estrogen and progesterone) at different times during the day. They focus their energies into finding the convenient one-a-day pill that contains everything for everyone.

A one-a-day pill might improve compliance, but the products I see in the marketing pipeline seem to be more unnatural than ever, making it even harder for a woman to adjust to her own individual needs.

Hormonal prescriptions are flawed unless they offer the exact replica of the hormone. If they fail to do that, I regard them as an insult to a woman's intelligence and her body.

I have four major objections to conventional estrogen prescriptions.

Objection 1: Are You a Horse? Do You Eat Hay? Why Take Horse Hormones?

The most widely used hormonal medications (such as Premarin, Premphase, and Prempro) contain so-called conjugated equine estrogens, estrogens extracted from the urine of a pregnant horse.

Does horse urine make horse sense for humans?

Show me the research glorifying a mare's urine over the urine of any other animal as the most effective source of estrogen replacement for the human female. A mare's urine contains a dozen different types of estrogen compounds. Only one of these compounds is an exact replica of one of your own estrogen compounds. The others are foreign.

I have never seen research proving that equine urine is the best source of estrogen for human females. In the absence of such research I can only suspect that the development of these products has something to do with the economics of horse urine. A mare is pregnant for a long time. A mare has a large bladder. And hay is cheap.

Why don't the drug companies extract the urine of teenaged females? Maybe create a nationwide system of hormone extraction based on urine collected from school rest rooms. Instead of allocating funds to schools from lotteries that encourage gambling, let the profits from this activity go back to the schools. Women would then have hormone replacements contributed by their fellow females instead of from horses.

As far-fetched as this notion sounds, it is not without precedence. Ancient Chinese physicians prepared potions from the urine of boys and girls to promote longevity and regenerate sexual vitality in both men and women.

Standard blood tests to measure your estrogen level are basically worthless if you take an equine-based estrogen replacement, including a new breed of prescriptions made from soy but still modeled on the equine formula. These formulas make it impossible to accurately determine your level of estrogen. You must wait at least eight weeks after stopping these medications before doing a blood test. Only after this period of time will the chemicalized estrogen be gone from your body.

Take the case of Dora, fifty-two, a short and full-breasted woman who came to see me—frustrated and confused. She had been started on Premarin by her physician and had been alarmed to see her breast size and weight increase substantially. Over the period of a year, her doctor increased the potency of her prescription three times. Each time she had been told that her estrogen blood level was still not high enough to give her the benefits.

Yet Dora had all the unmistakable signs of estrogen excess: painful, growing breasts, water retention, nervousness, and thirty pounds of unwanted weight.

Don't let anybody do this to you. Don't waste your time sitting for a blood test if you take estrogen from a horse. And if your body says you are taking enough estrogen, that should be the ultimate authority. Believe your body!

Objection 2: Fragmented Estrogen

Today we are seeing another huge distortion in the composition of conventional hormonal replacements. Many pills, patches, and injectibles generally contain only one human estrogen compound: estradiol (E2).

I have no idea why estradiol has been singled out, especially since we live in a time of estrogen dominance. So why give a woman an estrogen replacement containing only the most aggressive estrogen?

This contributes to many unnecessary side effects. In order to reduce the side effects, a new prescribing trend has emerged. Women are now put on lower and lower amounts of estrogen.

Moreover, physicians are now using bone density measurements as the sole determinant to calculate a patient's optimum intake of estrogen replacement. Estrogen prevents the loss of existing bone tissue. The problem with this approach is that lower estrogen intake can have the same protective effect on bone density as higher estrogen intake. But reduced intake will mean reduced estrogen benefits for the heart, brain, mood, feelings, sexuality, energy, sleep, and skin. Lower intake will not promote antiaging responses.

Pharmaceutical estradiol is a natural estrogen in the sense that it is an exact replica of the estradiol in our body, but it creates an overall hormonal imbalance and flies smack in the face of hormonal evolution. The primordial blueprint for estrogen in the human female is based on three compounds, not one. This is a holy hormonal trinity to be honored and maintained.

We have today the sophisticated scientific knowledge to extend a woman's life and to repair the damage that has been created from estrogen dominance. Women need balance more than ever in our modern age of birth control and estrogen proliferation. They don't need more imbalance.

We can take advantage of this opportunity by giving back to the body the perfect balance of estrogen compounds. The optimum balance is created with formulations that match the estrogen profile when a woman is pregnant. This means a balance high in protective estriol acting as a buffer against the excessive and aggressive estrogen compounds.

Objection 3: Deification and Misrepresentation of Soy Hormones

Hormone manufacturers are jumping on the "natural" bandwagon these days and trumpeting estrogen products made from soy and yams. But are they really natural? Let me take a moment here to focus on the soy example so that you can make informed choices.

Soy is a wonderful plant. We eat and enjoy many soy products, such as tofu, tempeh, miso, and soy milk. These products contain natural hormonelike compounds readily absorbed into the body. These compounds, known as phytoestrogens or isoflavones, go by the name of genistein, daidzein, and glycitein.

These isoflavones are weak chemicals, a thousand times weaker than the hormones in our bodies. When you eat soy, you assimilate these compounds. They get into your bloodstream and may generate some benefits. The benefits, however, are not nearly as significant as those that result from taking natural hormones.

The unique molecular structure of soy—and yams as well—has permitted scientists to readily extract from them the raw material that is processed through chemical reactions into the very same hormones in our body. For instance, all the three human estrogen compounds—estrone, estradiol, and estriol—are produced through this chemical process. So, too, are testosterone, DHEA, progesterone, and pregnenolone.

These exact replica hormones produced chemically are the hormones I use in my practice for my patients. They must, however, be identical to the hormones in the human body. If they are, they meet my criterion for natural.

Today, increasing numbers of pharmaceutical companies are producing hormonal products extracted from soy. These products are reconstituted in a way that is similar not to human estrogen but to equine urine estrogen. *The horse, it appears, has superseded the human as the pharmaceutical standard for estrogen!* Premarin has become the model hormone instead of a woman's own estrogen.

These products are then advertised as natural because they come from soy! The pharmaceutical companies can create any estrogen compound they want and yet they choose to follow the horse example.

I have seen advertisements for such products in medical journals showing a woman throwing her hands into the air in exaltation of nature. What is the difference here between estrogen extracted from a horse's urine or a soybean? There is no difference. Neither one belong in your body.

To me "natural" means to give to a woman's body what is natural to her body, whether you make it from soy, moonstone, or in the laboratory. If it is not the same, then it is foreign, no matter where it comes from. It is not part of the wholeness of the body's constitution. I regard it as an insult to a woman's intelligence to pawn off such unnatural natural products. A hormone made from soy or yam means nothing to me if it is anything less than an exact replica of the whole hormone that a woman has in her body.

Objection 4: Faulty Delivery

Estrogen replacement prescriptions deliver the hormone to your body via four forms: pills, patches, injections, and vaginal rings. They all have their problems.

Pills: First and foremost, estrogen pills cause the biggest increase of SHBG, resulting in the loss of benefits from other antiaging and essential hormones.

Oral estrogen stimulates another protein in the liver that raises blood pressure in about 8 percent of patients. I have seen this occur only once, however, among thousands of patients taking estrogen. In the one case, I eliminated the problem by switching the patient to an estrogen gel.

Another biochemical reaction from the liver is the production of a substance that could potentially increase blood-clotting activity. Any woman with a bleeding or clot-formation history should use only use the gel for this reason.

Oral estrogen may also slightly increase the risk of gallstones and insulin resistance. Any woman with hyperinsulinemia, prediabetes, or diabetes should avoid oral intake.

Patches: Pharmaceutical estrogen patches deliver a sustained, consistent release of the hormone into your body, without raising the sex hormone–binding globulin.

There are drawbacks, however. Patches contain only estradiol and thus carry the risk of creating a hormonal imbalance. Patch doses are fixed, and fixed doses are not appropriate when one accepts the premise that each individual may require different doses at different times. A woman cannot easily address daily or frequent fluctuations if she uses a fixed dose patch designed to last a week or two. And most women are fluctuating into the first five or ten years of menopause.

Patches often cause rashes on the body where applied. In one study, 24 percent of the participants experienced some type of skin reaction. The increasing availability of smaller patches makes this less of an annoyance.

An additional problem with patches is that they often don't stick to the skin and fall off prematurely.

If I use a pharmaceutical patch in my practice, I prefer Vivelle-Dot. It offers four dosage strengths, a smaller size, and appears to generate the least irritation. I use this product for patients who have used patches with satisfaction prior to seeing me and do not want to switch to natural hormones, or who have difficulty individualizing their dosage. In general, if you don't have access to natural hormones for whatever reason, use patches over pills, but avoid patches that combine estradiol with synthetic progesterone (progestins).

Injectibles: These products provide only estradiol, or estradiol derivatives, in a fixed dose. Given the normal state of fluctuations going on in the body, the dose may be too much or too little for what you need at a given time.

Vaginal administration (creams and vaginal rings): For years women were led to believe that when they use an estrogen cream vaginally, it doesn't affect them systemically. This is erroneous: significant absorption occurs systemically.

The advent of vaginal estrogen rings in recent years has offered a new and effective route for hormone delivery. They are designed to last for three months; however, in some cases they lose their potency earlier. Longer-lasting rings are now being developed.

Women often mention to me that they experience a constant pressure on the vagina from the ring. I am concerned that the presence of the ring might interfere with local lymphatic activity, that is, the network of vessels forming part of the body's defense system against infection. I am not aware, however, of any long-term side effects.

7

Basics of Natural Estrogen Replacement

The Benefits of Natural Estrogen Replacement

Estrogen is the starting point for restoring balance. I believe that natural estrogen can be supplemented with major antiaging and health benefits well before signs of significant deficiency develop. Estrogen replacement also can help those women who have had a suboptimal level throughout their reproductive years.

Here are some of the major dividends of estrogen replacement that I see among my patients, along with some typical comments:

- Control of mind and mood: "I can think clearly again."
- More stamina: "I can do more."

- Better sleep: "Finally, I don't wake up in the middle of the night anymore."
- Enhanced sense of femininity: "I care again about my body."
- Weight gain protection.
- Reduced risk of Alzheimer's disease, cardiovascular disease, bone loss, and arthritis.
- Maintenance of healthy skin: "My skin has regained its flush."
- Preservation of sexuality: "Sex is on my mind again."
- The breasts remain young and full: "It's as if my breast got a natural lift."
- Elimination of hot flashes and night sweats: "My thermostat works again."

Your Best Bet: Estrogen plus Progesterone

I prescribe natural estrogen along with natural progesterone. Progesterone is the evolutionary safeguard that enables you to enjoy the benefits of estrogen without side effects. It prevents an excess of estrogen buildup in the body. The two really go together.

In this section we will look at how to take and balance estrogen. Then, in part three, we will look at how to take and balance progesterone, as well as combine it with estrogen. In this sequential way, you will learn how to safely use these two primary hormones for maximum benefits.

Natural Estrogen Is a Prescription Item

All forms of natural estrogen that I recommend are available only through compounding pharmacies. You will need a doctor's prescription. Refer to my commentary in chapter 4 on making your physician your natural hormone therapy partner.

What Kind of Natural Estrogen Replacement Should You Take?

The basic natural estrogen formula I have used for years is *Tri-Estrogen,* or *Tri-Est,* for short. The formula was developed in the early 1980s by Jonathan Wright, M.D., an innovative Washington State physician who had been using estriol as an alternative to the conventional estrogen medications. He gradually realized that he could achieve maximum benefits by adding estradiol and estrone. To determine the best ratio of the three estrogen compounds, he measured blood and urinary levels. He found that a combination of 80 percent estriol, with 10 percent each of estradiol and estrone matched the body's own ratio. Other ratios might be more effective for certain conditions or at different times of a woman's life.

Wright is a clinician. I am a clinician. Physicians like us would love to be able to refer to research exploring the use of these natural compounds. Unfortunately, and amazingly, there is no such research. The financiers of medical research have no interest in natural hormones, only in altered, chemicalized substitutes that can be patented. From my clinical experience, Tri-Est works better for my patients than any pharmaceutical product. It is available in the following forms:

- capsules
- topical creams and gels
- sublingual drops
- vaginal creams
- suppositories
- troches (lozenges).

Tri-Est products are not available as patches.

Unlike pharmaceutical hormones, natural hormones are in and out of your body in eight to sixteen hours, and there is no cumulative effect.

I use different forms for different situations. *I generally see the best results with the gel.* However, some patients say the gel is messy or have some discomfort with it. There are other options that I will describe in this chapter. For many, convenience is as important a factor as effectiveness.

As you become more familiar with using hormones, keep in mind that there is no daily, weekly, or monthly formula for you to follow. You increase dosage when you need to increase, and you reduce dosage when you need to reduce. Until your body stops producing estrogen in menopause, the level is always fluctuating. Unfortunately, we don't have an "estrogenometer" that tells you how much your body is making every day. Sensing how you feel gives you the awareness of how much your body is using. Your awareness tells you when to go up or go down.

You may take the same amount for two months and feel great and then all of a sudden your breasts feel tender, you retain water, and you feel that there is something wrong with you.

There is nothing wrong with you. It's just that now your body is making more of the hormone on its own. So you reduce your replacement dosage.

I have had patients call and say, "Doctor Reiss, the hormone has worked for three months and now it isn't working at all."

"No," I say, "it's working. But now you need to take less . . . ."

Or more.

You get the point.

Just remember that your body will not mislead you. It will give you the signs. You just need to develop the confidence to recognize and believe what you are feeling. Always listen to your body. And always remember that your responses are going to be different from the next person because your physiology is different.

And don't forget what I mentioned earlier about the signs of estrogen deficiency and excess: *signs of deficiency are felt immediately. Signs of excess take longer.*

If I were to experimentally create an estrogen deficiency in a patient, she would develop hot flashes or mental fogginess immediately. If I were to give her too much estrogen, it would take a few days before we would see the changes, such as water retention, the breasts becoming fuller, and some snappy behavior.

For women who are very allergic, be aware of the possibility that an ingredient contained in a particular hormone product might cause a reaction. Such reactions are usually related to an oil or other substance used in the preparation that enhances its absorption in the body or delivery through the skin. The compounding pharmacist can replace these substances if they are problematic.

I have had only a few patients like this over the years. They were not able to use one particular form of hormone over a long period of time.

It is extremely unlikely that someone with a soy allergy would react to a natural hormone that was manufactured from soy. The reason is that there is none of the soy left in the end product, which is the pure hormone.

If you notice a skin rash as a result of using a hormonal gel, irritation in the vagina from a cream, gastrointestinal discomfort from a capsule, or a burning sensation of the tongue from sublingual drops, consider the following options:

- Switch the form of estrogen you use. Avoid what causes discomfort. You may have to use several different forms and alternate them on different days.
- Speak to a pharmacist at the compounding pharmacy where you obtained the product. I have found the pharmacists very professional, patient,

knowledgeable, and helpful. Discuss your individual needs with them. They can usually find a solution for you, such as changing a base ingredient that is part of the formula and helps deliver the hormone to the body. However, any change related to the hormone itself has to be authorized by your doctor. That includes changing the hormone strength.

Applying Estrogen Gel

Applied to the skin, estrogen gel offers excellent absorption, a relatively immediate effect, and maintains a consistent level of hormone in the body. It is diluted in the bloodstream before reaching the liver. Similar to pharmaceutical patches, this method of administration has the least influence on SHBG and, consequently, on other hormones. It avoids all the disadvantages of capsules that I will talk about in a moment.

When you apply the gel, rub it ten to fifteen times on any of the following parts of your body:

- The neck, the face, and brow. These locations yield the best absorption.
- The inner side of your upper right arm and forearm.
- The inner side of your upper left arm and forearm.

If you have any gel left over, rub it into the palms of your hands. Your abdomen or inner thighs are less ideal absorption sites.

Change locations frequently. Apply the gel over the widest surface as possible. Rub on the gel vigorously. You may notice a reddening of the skin afterward. This is a result of the blood vessels dilating from the rubbing action. The dilation effect is desirable. It increases the absorption.

Gel that contains alcohol should not be used vaginally. The alcohol can cause irritation of vaginal tissue. Nor should the gel be applied to the breasts or the nipples. Years ago I read a report that using the gel on nipples could significantly enhance their size. Some women might desire this effect. However, I do not know the long-term consequences and therefore cannot recommend it.

Ingredients used in gel products for delivering the hormone through the skin will probably vary among compounding pharmacies. If you are not getting the expected results with your gel, I suggest you may want to have your prescription filled at the pharmacies I have used for years. You will find them listed in Appendix A.

Most of the gel is absorbed within five to ten minutes. Always apply to a skin surface free of oils, moisturizers, or body lotions. These substances can interfere with absorption. It is best to use them about thirty minutes after the estrogen gel has been absorbed.

The gel you receive from the compounding pharmacy comes in a tube with a measuring device to help you gauge your dosage. Usually, after a few times, you will be able to squeeze out an appropriate amount onto your fingertip or a teaspoon without resorting to the device.

Individual dosing is quite easy because results are felt quickly, and in general last for about ten to sixteen hours, sometimes for as long as twenty-four hours. The natural hormone is in and out of your body within that time, unlike Premarin, the pharmaceutical estrogen, which generates effects for weeks or months.

Apply the gel twice a day—in the morning and before bedtime. I'll spell out the exceptions to this later as I discuss specific situations. In order to control their night sweats, some women apply more at bedtime than in the morning.

But anytime you need more, apply more. If you need less, apply less. *You will learn to know how much you need by how you feel.*

If you have signs of deficiency and feel your degree of improvement is not satisfactory, then simply increase your dosage, or reapply a partial dose an hour after the last application. You don't have to be uncomfortable and wait twelve hours. You can go up and down very easily with the gel in this manner and quickly become a master at individualizing your estrogen replacement to counteract your own hormonal fluctuations.

Let me share two examples to give you an idea of dosage manipulation.

Example 1

Joan, fifty-two, had been unable to fall asleep easily and suffered from night sweats, hot flashes, and a foggy mind. She applied 1 gram of the gel (a quarter teaspoon). She awoke the next morning feeling fresh, and her mind was somewhat clearer. She had slept better, yet still experienced some minimal hot flashes during the night.

The amount she initially took gave her significant but not quite enough relief. She still had some minimum problems. So in the morning she applied about 25 to 30 percent more of the gel. Throughout the day she felt excellent. Her mind was much clearer. In the evening she used the higher level of gel and had a smooth night.

Afterward, she continued with the same dose until she encountered signs of deficiency or excess. She learned to adjust upward or downward accordingly.

Example 2

Ruth, sixty, was feeling fine and had a lot of energy on $\frac{1}{2}$ gram of the gel (one-eighth of a teaspoon). However, she began to retain water and was having trouble putting on and taking off her rings. Her breasts had increased somewhat in size and become slightly tender to the touch.

At this point, Ruth's dosage was probably a bit too high for her. I told her to decrease the amount by a third. On the lowered dose, the problems cleared up.

Strength of Basic Gel

Each gram of the basic Tri-Est gel that I use contains 0.25 milligrams of estrone, 0.75 milligrams of estradiol, and 2.5 milligrams of estriol. A gram is equal to a quarter of a teaspoon.

When a potency problem arises with the use of a gel/cream, it could relate to the concentration of estrogen not being strong enough or not being well absorbed.

It you don't feel your prescription is strong enough, tell your doctor, who can then request a stronger potency for you.

Compounding pharmacists use different ingredients as bases and delivery agents for the hormone. As a result there can be a significant difference in effectiveness among prescriptions prepared by different pharmacies. I have found some prescriptions have as little as a quarter of the effectiveness of gels that I prescribe for my patients. If you have any doubts about effectiveness, ask the pharmacist to improve the delivery base ingredient of the formula or use the compounding pharmacists I recommend in Appendix A.

Taking Capsules

Capsules offer the most convenience. They may contain dry, micronized estrogen powder or powder dissolved in olive, safflower, sunflower, or peanut oil that act as "carriers" for the hormones. The best absorption occurs when you take the capsules with a meal that has some natural fat in it. The least effective absorption is on an empty stomach.

Taken orally, estrogen stimulates the liver to produce more HDL cholesterol, the so-called good cholesterol. Thus capsules can be beneficial for someone who needs to increase HDL. However, there's a potential downside here. Absorption through the oral route takes estrogen quickly to the liver, which then releases sex hormone–binding insulin. I described the negative impact of this scenario earlier, in chapter 5.

Another problem, at least for a small percentage of women, is that oral estrogen can unleash a chemical in the body that causes hot flashes. For these women, the reaction can occur both with patented, chemicalized hormone substitutes or natural estrogen. Since hot flashes are a sign of deficiency, you and your physician may think you are still low on estrogen despite taking the hormone. Sometimes doctors will give a patient more estrogen, yet the hot flashes will continue, and signs of excess estrogen may develop.

Capsules can be customized to include a variety of hormones. This is handy for someone wishing to take several hormones at one time, and who is hormonally stable without bothersome fluctuations. I would recommend estrogen in a separate capsule, however, if you are dealing with a lot of fluctuations. And overall, the absorption of hormones combined in one capsule is not as good as if they are taken individually.

Strength of Capsules

The strength of the standard Tri-Est estrogen capsules ranges from 0.625 to 2.5 milligrams. The lower-dose capsule contains 0.0625 milligrams of estrone, 0.0625 milligrams of estradiol, and 0.5 milligrams of estriol.

Taking Sublingual Drops

Drops are also very convenient and, in addition, make the process of increasing or decreasing dosage quite simple.

Estrogen sublingual drops are quickly absorbed. The results are felt immediately. Don't swallow the drops. Simply apply them under the tongue. To speed absorption, wiggle your tongue back and forth.

I recommend sublingual drops in the following situations:

- If you need estrogen *intermittently.* That means you don't need it on a daily basis or perhaps only a few days out of the cycle.
- To help with the *wide fluctuations of perimenopause,* where you may need a small amount one day but much more the following day.
- For the *relief of migraines* that are estrogen-related. Are you aware that many more women than men suffer from migraines? Estrogen is a major reason. A woman with migraines can use the sublingual drops three or four times a day in order to create an even level of estrogen. A few drops can also be taken at the first sign of a migraine.

Sublingual drops quickly introduce a high tide of estrogen into the body. The level falls relatively fast afterward. Usually after twelve hours little is left. Some people need to repeat the application three or four times a day.

I find that about 70 percent of women who use sublingual drops daily (especially those who use more than three drops twice a day) also increase their SHBG level. Even though the hormone is absorbed into the bloodstream and doesn't go directly to the liver, as is the case with capsules, the liver tends to overreact to the sudden rise in estrogen. When this occurs, I recommend switching to another form of estrogen.

To enhance palatability, you can request the compounding pharmacist who prepares your prescription to flavor them. Among my patients, orange and mint are popular flavors.

Strength of Sublingual Drops

Ask for Tri-Est drops with the same potency as the capsules, that is, each drop contains 0.625 milligrams of estrogen. Thus, each drop delivers 0.0625 milligrams of estrone (E1), 0.0625 of estradiol (E2), and 0.5 milligrams of estriol (E3). You can also order a higher concentration if that is more convenient for you.

In my guidelines in the following chapters, I recommend taking a certain number of drops. *Please don't confuse drops with dropperfuls.* A dropperful gives you too many drops, many more than you would want to take at one time.

Some women become quite cavalier about the number of drops they use. As a result they take more than they need. My advice is to learn to recognize the level in the dropper that relates to your dosage. If you take three drops, see what three drops look like in the dropper. Just a moment or two of experimenting with the dropper will enable you to more precisely eyeball your appropriate dosage. If you try to feel the falling drops under your tongue you will probably take more than you intend.

Using Vaginal Creams (or Gels without Alcohol)

Estrogen creams are applied vaginally. Absorption is excellent. In my practice I use estrogen creams to help restore proper vaginal elasticity and lubrication, as well as promote better urinary tract function. For the great majority of patients, I recommend estriol (E3) alone. Estriol, you will remember, is the least aggressive and most protective of the three estrogen compounds.

When you use estrogen systemically (capsules, sublingual drops or topical gels, both pharmaceutical and natural), *about 30 percent of women do not expe-*

rience the desired degree of vaginal benefits. For these individuals, the addition of the cream can make a big difference.

Over the years I have observed patients making two major errors regarding the use of vaginal estrogen creams:

Error 1: They apply vaginal creams on the skin. These creams are poorly absorbed through the skin and should only be used vaginally.

Error 2: Some women who want to avoid any method that carries estrogen into the body systemically, mistakenly choose a vaginal cream. They believe the cream acts only locally to enhance vaginal functionality without absorption to the rest of the body. The vagina is indeed an excellent absorption site for estrogen, but it's also a gateway to the body beyond.

Strength of Creams

One gram of cream contains 1 to 2 milligrams of estriol.

Taking Troches (Lozenges) or Sublingual Pills

Troches can be either chewed or sucked. However, I do not recommend them or sublingual pills.

These forms nearly always increase the SHBG level and do not lend themselves to adjusting dosages readily. They have the disadvantages of the capsules and drops, without any of their redeeming advantages.

Substitutes for Natural Estrogen

Some of my patients refuse to take estrogen. Some say they don't want to alter the course of the aging process. Others are influenced by the media reports that have put so much fear into the hearts of women throughout our society.

Yet many of these women are keenly interested in decreasing the symptoms of estrogen deficiency with alternative methods.

The first alternative is to take estriol alone. Although this is one of the estrogen compounds, scientific data repeatedly singles out this constituent for its protective role against breast cancer.

Estriol will enhance vaginal lubrication and elasticity, prevent night sweats and hot flashes, and promote the health of the skin. It will also somewhat improve mental clarity. My recommendation is 2 to 7 milligrams of estriol twice a day in the form of capsules or drops. Estriol alone, just as with all other estrogens, must be taken with progesterone. I will describe how to combine the two later.

For a woman who will not consider estriol, the following supplement and food options may be helpful:

- **Black cohosh.** This herb is said to reduce hot flashes. I regard this as putting a Band-Aid over a wound. The lessening of hot flashes, while desirable, does not restore estrogen balance.
- **Dong quai (Chinese angelica).** This popular "female remedy" herb is suggested for painful periods, vaginal dryness, and menopause-related changes. In menopause, the herb reduces the level of estrogen. For this reason I do not recommend it for menopausal women.
- **Extracts of pomegranates and red clover.** You are fooling yourself thinking you are not ingesting estrogen. Pomegranates and red clover contain estrogen compounds, and that is why you may experience some relief. But it makes more sense to me to use a measurable amount of your identical hormone, obtainable from a compounding pharmacy, than to take a product that gives you no reliable levels or quality.
- **Soy and yams.** Eating large amount of soy products, as is common in the Orient, can reduce subjective signs of estrogen deficiency in many women, including night sweats, hot flashes, and vaginal dryness.

    Taking soy supplements, which contain phytoestrogens called isoflavones, can also be helpful for some women. I have found they give significant relief for about 25 percent of the individuals who take them.

    You need 50 to 150 milligrams of isoflavones daily. The isoflavone ratio should be 50 percent genistein, 40 percent daidzein, and 10 percent glycitein.

    Eating yams will not achieve relief of estrogen symptoms. Although estrogen and other hormones are chemically extracted from yams, your body cannot utilize the hormones they contain *as* hormones when you eat yams or yam extracts.
- **Maca.** Sometimes referred to as Peruvian ginseng, this highland plant has long been a source of food and healing to the Andean Indians. Among its many medicinal applications, the dried maca root is promoted for relief of menopausal changes. As a supplement, I have seen it help about 25 percent of the women who use it. Those who do receive benefits may experience some breast tenderness. Advocates of maca do not recommend the herb for individuals with a high risk or history of breast cancer.

WHAT TO DO NOW

In this chapter I have given you both general and practical information on estrogen and estrogen products. This is knowledge you need to help you make informed decisions. In the following chapters, I will give you specifics—when, how, in what form, and how much of natural estrogen to administer for menopause (including surgical menopause resulting from removal of ovaries), perimenopause, and for younger women.

Even though the next chapter deals with menopause, it also provides other important information—like the "Estrogen Quick Check"—that all women using this book should read.

8

Natural Estrogen Replacement for Menopause

WHAT'S IN THIS CHAPTER

- Defining menopause
- The three categories of menopause: onset, mid-menopause, late menopause
- Menopausal women with no symptoms
- The goal of natural estrogen replacement
- Before starting natural estrogen
- Natural estrogen for onset menopause
- Natural estrogen in mid-menopause
- Natural estrogen in late menopause
- What if you have had a hysterectomy
- What if your ovaries were removed
- What if your ovaries were affected by chemotherapy
- Monitoring your intake—the "Estrogen Quick Check"
- Dose adjustment scenarios
- Monitoring your intake with your physician

Defining Menopause

Women typically associate menopause with night sweats, hot flashes, and the end of menstruation. According to the North American Menopause Society, most women in the industrialized world experience natural menopause at about age fifty-one, but it can occur in the thirties and more rarely as late as in the late fifties. From the medical standpoint, menopause is said to become "official" when a woman goes without a menstrual period for twelve straight months.

To me, menopause is not about having or not having a period. Young women can stop having periods because they are anorexic, lose too much weight, or are involved in intense athletic activity. They are not in menopause. Some women never have periods. Their endocrine systems fail to mature and they require medical treatment. They are not menopausal either.

I associate menopause with *persistent signs of estrogen deficiency*. In my determination of menopause, I consider both subjective and objective confirmations. The criteria include:

1. **Subjective signs of estrogen deficiency.** Refer to the beginning of chapter 5.
2. **Laboratory tests to confirm deficiency.** These following tests can help guide you—and your physician—in choosing the most effective form of estrogen.

   - **Estradiol (E2).** A low level of estradiol (under 40 pg/ml), along with a high FSH level, suggests menopause.
   - **FSH.** Follicle-stimulating hormone acts as the messenger for the pituitary gland (the body's master gland), which commands the ovaries to produce estrogen. During perimenopause and menopause, as ovarian production of estrogen decreases, the body releases more FSH in an effort to stimulate the ovaries. In menopause, the FSH level tops 20 miu/ml and often soars to over 100. High FSH and low estradiol inform us that the body is trying hard but failing to stimulate estrogen production.
   - **SHBG.** An optional test is to measure the level of the sex hormone–binding globulin, which I discussed at length in chapter 5. I always measure the baseline value of SHBG prior to treatment. This provides a major biochemical marker for comparison after estrogen replacement is started.

3. **Pelvic ultrasound.** This procedure provides an anatomical confirmation of menopause. It gives a visual record of the state of the uterus lining and ovaries. Usually in menopause, we see a thin endometrium (the lining of the uterus) and ovaries that appear small and atrophied. Ultrasound is becoming an integral aspect of pelvic examinations and is commonly available in physicians' offices.

The Three Categories of Menopause

In order to calculate your starting point for natural hormone replacement, we need to first fit you into one of three general categories of menopause: onset, mid, or late. Each stage typically has a different intensity of estrogen fluctuations and requires different dosing in order to achieve maximum benefits.

If you are not a perfect fit for one particular group, you will at least have a general idea. Keep in mind that some women don't experience major fluctuations at all.

1. Onset Menopause

This category refers to the first few years of menopause, where women still experience large fluctuations from time to time, yet less frequently than during perimenopause. There is no menstrual cycle. Prior to estrogen replacement, the symptoms of deficiency are at their peak.

I have successfully treated many women in this stage of menopause with natural hormones who were in an extreme state of physiological distress. They were often out of control, having difficulty sleeping, and concentrating, and otherwise carrying out the normal activities of life.

It is this group of women that I have found to be the most enthusiastic about balancing their hormones and prolonging their feminine youthfulness.

2. Mid-menopause

This category refers to the next five years of menopause, that is, women who are three to eight years into the change.

Estrogen fluctuations still occur; however, they are minimal. For individuals not on hormone replacement, there is a significant reduction of some symptoms of estrogen deficiency, especially night sweats and hot flashes.

Many women who are not taking hormones interpret the absence of night sweats and hot flashes as an indication that they are no longer in menopause. They will tell me that "I am postmenopausal" or "I am no longer in menopause." Not so. All it means is that they don't have night sweats and hot flashes. They still have most of the signs of estrogen deficiency. Either they have learned to live with these symptoms or are taking medication for them, such as antidepressants, sleeping pills, tranquilizers, and vaginal lubricants.

In my clinic I don't use the term "postmenopausal." I really don't know what it means. Is a woman who becomes menopausal one day considered postmenopausal the day after? If she has no more hot flashes or night sweats does that mean she is postmenopausal? To me, a woman who becomes menopausal is menopausal for the rest of her life.

3. Late Menopause

This group generally includes women over sixty. They have been in menopause for ten to fifteen years or more. There have been barely any fluctuations in their estrogen.

It is never too late to start estrogen. Even a woman in her eighties can experience estrogen benefits to the bones, heart, vagina, skin, breasts, mind, mood, and overall well-being.

Menopausal Women with No Symptoms

Some women breeze through menopause, experiencing some loss of breast fullness, dryness of the vagina, and wrinkling of the skin, but none of the changes that make life miserable for many others. Such women often have functioned on a relatively low level of estrogen throughout their lives. For them, now in menopause, the hormonal decline is not significant enough to cause problems.

For other women, there is no loss of breast fullness, vaginal functionality, or vitality of the skin. Their estrogen levels are higher in relation to other women in menopause. Some of them also are able to readily convert other hormones—such as the testosterone and DHEA present in their body—into estrogen. This cellular process is known as aromatization. Despite the name, this process has nothing to do with smell.

There is a reason for concern here. The relatively higher level of estrogen at this stage of life implies the existence of estrogen dominance. Remember, there is no progesterone in the body to balance the estrogen. In medical terms, we say the estrogen is "unopposed." We have to be alert to a potentially threatening imbalance that could lead to endometrial cancer and negative long-term effects on a woman's health.

If you are in this situation, I suggest you see your gynecologist or primary care physician for a pelvic ultrasound and estrogen blood level test. If the ultrasound is negative, meaning there is no thickening of the endometrium, there may be no need to worry. A thickening of tissue, caused by the "unopposed" estrogen, should be evaluated further, as this could possibly be a precancerous condition. It is definitely in your best interest to take proper precautions. That includes a checkup and *progesterone replacement to balance your estrogen.*

The Goal of Natural Estrogen Replacement

My goal is to restore the whole range of functions and benefits that are lost with estrogen deficiency. This is a very different approach than conventional medicine, which, in my opinion, focuses erroneously on one measurement: restoring bone mineral density.

The medical indication for most of the hormonal medications receiving FDA approval for use in menopause relates to preventing osteoporosis. This has become the major criterion. Pharmaceutical companies are developing new generations of prescriptions containing the lowest level of estrogen necessary to create an accepted degree of bone density improvement. *This single-minded approach inflates the bone issue, and ignores the many other estrogen-related issues that make a woman a woman—such as intelligence, sensuality, and emotions.*

It's as if they are saying:

"You are just your bones, forget your womanhood."
"If you are depressed, no problem, we have antidepressants for you."
"If you can't sleep, we have sleeping pills."
"If you have anxiety, we have tranquilizers."
"If your skin sags, we can stretch it."
"If you gain weight, we have weight loss pills or can suck the fat out."
"If your breasts are falling, we have the Wonder Bra."
"If you have migraines, we have migraine pills."

Estrogen replacement must be seen in a broader concept that goes beyond bones. An optimum replacement for each woman can resolve the major and minor problems associated with deficiency and reroute the whole body onto a healthy and youthful U-turn.

Even an eighty-year-old woman can feel beautiful and sensual again, be proud of her body, and improve her clarity of mind. She can often restore the femininity lost with the years of estrogen depletion.

Before Starting Natural Estrogen

I recommend five preliminary steps before starting on natural estrogen. These are medical tests and exams you will need to discuss with your physician.

1. Check the estradiol (E2) level for an estrogen baseline. If you are currently using an equine form of estrogen (Premarin-type products) or a soy product based on the equine formula, you have to wait at least eight weeks after you stop taking them before testing. These compounds, for reasons I explained in chapter 6, give false estrogen readings.

2. Check the level of SHBG to further determine estrogen status.
3. For women presumably in the early stage of menopause, check the FSH level to confirm the diagnosis of menopause. Many patients have come to me over the years who were previously prescribed a variety of unnecessary estrogen treatments because they were thought to be in menopause. When I evaluated their situation, I found they were not, in fact, in menopause.
4. A recent physical and gynecological checkup, breast exam, mammogram, and Pap smear.
5. Pelvic ultrasound to learn the status of the endometrium. Any suspicious condition should be dealt with in a timely manner. This also avoids natural estrogen replacement being cited as the cause for an otherwise pre-existing condition.

Natural Estrogen for Onset Menopause

The earlier you are in menopause, the more reactions to estrogen fluctuations you are likely to feel. You may experience dramatic differences, as many women do, from one day to the next, one week to the next, or one month to the next. While the overall amount of estrogen your body produces is decreasing, it will generally not bottom out until you are in menopause for several years.

You can assess the degree of fluctuations by how you feel prior to starting any hormonal replacement program. Significant fluctuations translate to a lot of emotional and physical turbulence. This means you are likely to require more self-adjusting of your estrogen replacement.

Minor discomfort translates to minor fluctuations. This means you probably won't need frequent adjusting of your dosage.

Always keep in mind that the estrogen you take in your hormonal replacement program is not the only estrogen you have. Your body is still producing estrogen. And because of that you may have to compensate, and increase or decrease your dosage. How often you change is a totally individual matter. Some women may have to readjust every few days in the beginning, some every few months, others every few years. Some may not need to change at all.

Don't be afraid to experience the ups and downs and how they affect you. Just stay in tune with your body. The changes you feel will give you the cues to learn the personal art of fine-tuning and optimum balance.

In general, you'll be taking the same amount of estrogen twice a day, morning and evening. I find that this approach works well for about 90 per-cent of my patients.

The exceptions are as follows:

* Women who feel they don't need a second dose in the evening. For them, the single morning dose works fine.

I should point out, however, that after sixteen hours the estrogen replacement level in the body falls significantly. Even though you may not experience symptoms of deficiency when the level goes down, I would prefer you try to take a second dose, even if it is smaller than the first. The reason is that you will then receive the full protective benefits of estrogen—for the heart, bones, and nervous system—around the clock.

If you try a second dose of any quantity and develop any signs of excess estrogen, then just stick with the one dose. For a small percentage of indi-viduals, one dose a day is enough to maintain an adequate level of estrogen for twenty-four hours.

* Some women cannot tolerate a full dose in the evening but are able to take a smaller dose.
* Some women need to take more in the evening than the morning in order to eliminate severe night sweats.
* Some women need to take estrogen more than twice a day.

Guidelines for Starting Estrogen for Onset Menopause

Gel. Begin with ½ gram (one-eighth of a teaspoon) of the basic Tri-Est gel twice a day. Each gram contains 0.25 milligrams of estrone, 0.75 milligrams of estradiol, and 2.5 milligrams of estriol.

Whenever you need to increase dosage, do so by ¼ of a gram, that is, one-sixteenth of a teaspoon. The average range is ¼ gram to 1½ grams each time.

If you need to decrease, do it the same way—by increments of ¼ of a gram.

Capsules. Start with the basic Tri-Est 0.625 milligram capsule, containing 0.0625 milligrams of estrone (E1), 0.0625 milligrams of estradiol (E2), and 0.5 milligrams of estriol (E3).

Take two capsules twice a day. Then increase or decrease as needed. Do not exceed a total of six capsules at a time. Anytime you require more, your situation needs to be reevaluated by your physician.

If you find you are doing well and are using a consistent number of capsules, you may want to contact the compounding pharmacy that filled your prescription and request a more concentrated dosage. In other words, take fewer pills that give you the same amount. Your compounding pharmacist can help you streamline the process with your physician's approval.

Here are some examples:

- If you take two Tri-Est 0.625-milligram capsules twice a day, you may want to switch to one Tri-Est capsule of 1.25 milligrams twice a day.
- If you take three Tri-Est 0.625-milligram capsules twice a day, you may want to consolidate to one Tri-Est capsule at 1.75-milligram strength twice a day.
- If you take four of the Tri-Est 0.625-milligram capsules twice a day, you may want to choose one capsule with 2.25 milligrams twice a day.

Anytime you make such changes, be sure to hang on to your remaining .625 capsules. Estrogen fluctuations are unpredictable. The smaller-dose capsules will be handy if you want to increase or decrease your dosage with a smaller increment.

What if you need to increase your capsule dosage? With your estrogen level falling over the months and years, you may well come to the time when you need to increase your dosage.

If you have regularly used the Tri-Est 1.25- or 1.75-milligram strength capsule twice daily, initially add a Tri-Est 0.625-milligram capsule once or twice daily as needed. Wait until you feel stable again. Then ask your physician to contact your compounding pharmacist to formulate another capsule that meets your changing needs.

If you are using a Tri-Est 1.25-milligram capsule twice daily, you can also try to double up once or twice a day. Don't try to double up on the higher Tri-Est 1.75- or 2.25-milligram strength capsules. You may wind up taking too much estrogen as a result.

What if you need to decrease your capsule dosage? If you experience signs of excess estrogen and are using the higher strength Tri-Est capsules, simply skip one of the daily doses for a day or two.

If it seems that you are in a period where you need less estrogen for more than a few days, start to decrease your dosage by using a reduced-strength capsule. For instance, instead of a single Tri-Est 2.25-milligram capsule, take a 1.75-milligram capsule; instead of a 1.75-milligram capsule, take a 1.25 capsule.

Sublingual drops. This form is extremely easy to use and achieve balance, especially for individuals who still experience frequent fluctuations.

Start with one or two drops of Tri-Est 0.625-milligram strength twice daily. The maximum is six for any single dosage at this strength. If you need to take more, you require a reevaluation.

Guidelines for Switching from Pharmaceutical Estrogen

If you take 0.625-milligram strength Premarin, Premphase, Prempro, or Estratab, or 1-milligram strength Estrace, or use patches with 0.05-milligram strength, start with the following amounts of natural estrogen:

Gel: 1/2 to 3/4 gram of the basic Tri-Est gel twice daily (one-eighth to one-sixteenth of a teaspoon). Each gram of the basic gel contains a combination of 0.25 milligrams of estrone, 0.75 milligrams of estradiol, and 2.5 milligrams of estriol. Remember that absorption may vary due to the type of base ingredients used in the formula for delivering the hormone into the body.

Capsules. One Tri-Est 1.25-milligram strength capsule or two 0.625-milligram capsules twice daily.

Sublingual drops. One or two drops twice daily.

If you take 1.25-milligram strength Premarin, Premphase, Prempro, or Estratab, or 2-milligram strength Estrace, or use patches with .1-milligram strength, start with the following amounts of natural estrogen:

Gel. 1 gram of the basic Tri-Est gel twice daily (one-quarter teaspoon).

Capsules. One 2.25-milligram strength Tri-Est capsule twice daily.

Sublingual drops. Four drops twice daily.

Natural Estrogen in Mid-Menopause

Usually there are fewer fluctuations in this stage of menopause. They may come on suddenly and unexpectedly, and they are sometimes associated with the formation of benign ovarian cysts. You can generally achieve balance quite readily at this stage.

Some women who start to take estrogen at mid-menopause experience hot flashes or night sweats again, and naturally they become upset. Before the estrogen replacement they no longer had any problems. Now they do. The reason is that the "thirst" for estrogen was revived.

I believe that when you stop having hot flashes, the body in essence has given up reminding you of its need for estrogen. Yet the body never loses its desire for estrogen. The moment you reintroduce estrogen, the incredible sensor in the body is reawakened that tells you how much you need.

When this occurs, raise your estrogen intake to the needed level. The hot flashes or night sweats should disappear. You can use the disappearance of symptoms as a guide for achieving an appropriate estrogen level.

Guidelines for Starting in Mid-Menopause

Gel. Start with 1 gram (one-quarter of a teaspoon) of the basic Tri-Est gel twice daily. One gram of the basic gel contains 0.25 milligrams of estrone, 0.75 milligrams of estradiol, and 2.5 milligrams of estriol.

Capsules. Start with the basic Tri-Est 0.625-milligram capsule. Take three or four capsules twice a day. Or two Tri-Est 1.25-milligram strength capsules twice daily.

Sublingual drops. Start with three or four drops twice daily. Usually you will attain balance fairly quickly.

Guidelines for Switching from Pharmaceutical Estrogen

Follow the same instructions as for onset menopause.

Natural Estrogen in Late Menopause

Older women require a very conservative approach. Any minor reaction, such as slight breast tenderness, a tiny pimple, or an alteration in skin tone, can be very unsettling.

I often start older patients with other hormones, such as DHEA or human growth hormones, before using estrogen. When I do add estrogen I use a much lower dose than for younger women and I increase the amount very slowly. Older women have less estrogen. That doesn't mean they need a higher dosage.

Anytime a hormone replacement program is started, whether a female is twenty-one or ninety-one, the possibility exists that some uterine bleeding could develop, the result of sloughing of the uterine lining. Cramping might precede any bleeding. A low-dose approach usually minimizes the chance of bleeding, which can be so unsettling to a woman in her seventies or beyond.

Although the bleeding usually stops within a few weeks, be sure to inform the physician who is monitoring you.

If the bleeding is accompanied by signs of excess estrogen, such as breast tenderness or water retention, that's a message telling you to decrease the amount of estrogen you are taking.

Be sure also to have an ultrasound prior to estrogen replacement. Don't compromise on this. A good number of women in late menopause have had a small degree of unopposed estrogen for some time. As a result they may have developed an endometrial tissue overgrowth. Some may even have asymptomatic cancer of the uterus. A simple ultrasound will provide you and your physician with an accurate picture of the status of your uterine lining.

At this menopausal stage, a woman should have an endometrial lining less than three millimeters thick. Even the five-millimeter standard considered normal is a bit too thick.

Guidelines for Starting in Late Menopause

Gel. Start with ½ gram (one-eighth of a teaspoon) of a weaker Tri-Est gel containing 0.1 milligram of estrone (E1), 0.1 milligram of estradiol (E2), and 1 milligram of estriol (E3). Apply twice daily. You can obtain this diluted formula from a compounding pharmacy. In a month, you can increase the dosage to a full gram twice a day. This amount is still much less than the full-strength gel.

If you wish to increase further, obtain a higher strength Tri-Est formula containing 0.2 milligram of estrone, 0.2 milligram of estradiol, and 2 milligrams of estriol in ½ gram of gel. Apply ½ gram twice a day. In another month, you can increase to a full gram of this compound twice a day if you desire.

Capsules. Start with one basic Tri-Est 0.625-milligram capsule once a day. After a few weeks, take one capsule twice a day. Every few weeks you can increase the number of capsules, as long as you are comfortable. Don't exceed three capsules twice daily. If you reach that level, you may want to request the compounding pharmacy to make a stronger potency capsule for you, so that you take fewer pills. For instance, you could consolidate your dosage into one Tri-Est 1.25- or 1.75-milligram capsule twice a day.

Most women eventually take between one Tri-Est 0.625- or 1.75-milligram capsule twice daily.

Guidelines for Switching from Pharmaceutical Estrogen

Follow the same guidelines as for onset menopause.

If you have been taking pharmaceutical estrogen, your body is accustomed to a higher level of estrogen.

What If You Have Had a Hysterectomy?

Premenopausal removal of the uterus is not a ticket to menopause. Yet many studies show that estrogen production decreases frequently after surgery even though the ovaries are still intact. As a result, subjective signs of estrogen deficiency associated with menopause may develop. I have seen this many times among new patients.

Today, most women with hysterectomies are conventionally treated with estrogen alone. In one sense they are lucky. They have not been exposed to the potential harm of chemicalized progestins that are part of the standard combined hormonal replacement program.

I believe, however, they should not be denied the benefits of *natural progesterone* when they start hormonal replacement therapy. For details on how to do that, refer to chapter 14.

To start natural estrogen, follow the guidelines for the onset menopause group.

What If Your Ovaries Were Removed?

Premenopausal surgery to remove the ovaries leads directly and immediately to full menopause. The body's main source of estrogen (as well as progesterone and testosterone) is eliminated in one surgical stroke.

A woman facing oophorectomy should always discuss hormonal replacement treatment with her physician prior to surgery. At that point, and not afterward, she should make an informed decision about what type of replacement program she wishes to follow. She should have the replacement hormones on hand and start them immediately after surgery.

What If Your Ovaries Were Damaged by Chemotherapy?

Chemotherapy of any type has the potential to damage the ovaries at any age and trigger an abrupt drop in estrogen production. The effect could be minimal and not disturb ovarian function. It could be temporary. But it could even throw a woman into permanent menopause.

If the disturbance is significant, you will need to replace the lost estrogen. My recommendation is the gel form. You want to reduce any possible burden on the liver, even minimal, that might occur from using either capsules or sublingual drops.

Start with a relatively high dose of estrogen, the same level as the mid-menopause starting group.

If the ovaries recover their normal function after a period of time, and return to making estrogen again, you may start to notice symptoms of estrogen excess. Reduce your intake of estrogen replacement as needed to eliminate any symptoms. If the recovery is complete, you may need to stop estrogen.

But be alert for signs of deficiency after you reduce or stop the estrogen. And, if need be, resume the estrogen at whatever level it takes to prevent the new symptoms.

Monitoring Your Intake—the Estrogen Quick Check

The following four-point routine can help you quickly determine if you are taking too much or too little estrogen. Use it twice a day, before you take estrogen, and for as long as you experience symptoms of hormonal fluctuations. It only takes a moment or two.

Once you reach a stable level and take the same basic dosage of estrogen most of the time, then there is no need to use this routine. Refer back to it anytime you feel out of balance and want to adjust your intake.

As you perform this simple routine, always keep your individuality in mind. Not everyone experiences all the typical hormonal-related changes. You may feel hot flashes, or have difficulty falling asleep, or experience mental fogginess or depression. Or you may get the full brunt—all the discomfort.

And remember that there are a minority of women—about 5 percent—who feel no changes whatsoever, regardless of whether they have too little or too much estrogen.

Dose Adjustment Scenarios

Use the following examples as further guides to help learn how to self-adjust your dosage of estrogen. In my clinical experience, it doesn't take my patients very long before they are quite familiar with their own reactions and how to interpret them for optimum effect. I am sure you will become readily adept as well.

Example 1

You wake up feeling a bit foggy. You didn't sleep well. You had hot flashes and night sweats. Your breasts feel normal. You are not very enthusiastic about facing the upcoming activities of the day. You feel low.

Here's what to do:

If you took two Tri-Est 0.625-milligram capsules the night before, you should now increase the dosage. Add one capsule in the morning.

THE ESTROGEN QUICK CHECK

1. The Breast Check

Touch and feel your breasts.

If they are full, painful, or growing, that generally indicates too much estrogen.

If they have lost some of their fullness, or seem to be dropping, that means more estrogen is needed.

The status of the breasts can be used as a yardstick for individualizing your dosage of estrogen replacement. Increase when your breasts are not full. Decrease if they are enlarged or painful.

These basic criteria will serve you well, provided you also take enough progesterone.

Women with breast implants cannot use this test to assess their estrogen dosage.

2. The Ring Check

Do you wear rings? How easy are they to slip on and off?

Difficulty removing rings generally indicates too much estrogen. If the rings move easily then your level is correct.

3. The Sleep Check

How are you sleeping?

If you have difficulty falling asleep, or experience restless nights, you might not have enough estrogen. If you awake drenched in perspiration, your estrogen level is very low. You need more. If you experience minimum hot flashes, your level is still not optimum. Take slightly more than you took the night before.

4. Mind and Mood Check

For many women, mental clarity and mood are extremely accurate measurements of estrogen replacement. Others, however, may find the mental and mood signs too subtle or overlapping to use as effective indicators.

Not enough estrogen. Is your mind a little foggy in the morning? Are you feeling a little down? Confused? Not in good control of your mood? Don't care how you look? Your level may be lower than optimum. Take more than you took the night before.

Too much estrogen. Are you feeling uptight? Irritated? But your mind is clear? Your level may be too high. Decrease the amount.

The two capsules are equal to two 0.625 Tri-Est sublingual drops or ½ gram of the standard Tri-Est gel (containing 0.25 milligrams of E1, 0.75 milligrams of E2, and 2.5 milligrams of E3). If you are using the drops, add one drop in the morning. If you are using the gel, use an additional 25 to 50 percent more gel, in the morning.

The beauty of this approach is that the response is fairly immediate, particularly with the drops and the gel. You will feel the effect within a half hour to two hours. With the capsules, give it two hours.

If you increase the dose and feel better, but yet not quite tip-top, you might increase the dosage a bit more. You don't have to wait a full twelve hours in discomfort. Refer back to my general guidelines on using the different forms of estrogen in chapter 7.

Example 2

You wake up after a good night's sleep but feel a bit uptight, with slight breast tenderness and swelling in your fingers. Those are signs indicating you should take less today than you did the night before.

The estrogen effect on the mood, clarity of the mind, hot flashes, and the desire to be sensual is quite immediate for most women. But don't expect to see water retention and breast tenderness resolve overnight. These symptoms take a few days.

Bottom line. Achieving your optimum dosage means paying attention to your body. You must know your body and your reactions. Learn the signs and adjust accordingly. It's not difficult. Your body is your yardstick.

Please remember your individuality. You might have unique responses that I haven't mentioned. Use them in your fine-tuning process.

Your ability to sense changes is also very individual. Some changes may be very subtle and more difficult to assess. Don't be discouraged. Just remember that only you can make the determination. Nobody else can do it for you and say this or that is a good dose for you—not me, not the pharmacist, not your doctor. Only your body can tell you.

The most important yardstick is how you feel. I have learned from the thousands of women I help care for and monitor personally that if you feel well you are probably taking a correct dosage.

Monitoring Your Intake with Your Physician

It is still very prudent to work with your physician to monitor your progress. Most patients feel comfortable having an objective medical test to measure the level of estrogen in their body. Never consider yourself definitively adjusted without the backup of proper medical monitoring.

Reading Blood Tests

I monitor patients by checking their blood estradiol (E2) level. Blood tests are far from perfect, but basically they assure me that a patient isn't taking far too much or far too little hormone.

I tend to rely more on the tests in difficult cases. These involve situations where I cannot easily assess whether a patient is taking too much or not enough estrogen. The tests also help in those very rare cases where patients take a very large or very small dose without showing signs of excess or deficiency.

I compare blood findings to the subjective feedback from a patient. How you feel reflects the action of the hormone at the cellular level, that is, how it is doing its job and impacting cells. There are no tests to monitor that. Your cellular response is an individual matter. One woman may be stable at 50 pg/ml of estrogen while another may require 200 pg/ml, a fourfold difference, to feel balanced.

Generally, there will be many fluctuations if you are early on in menopause. Remember that you also have your own estrogen production operating in your body. You haven't stopped producing. Whatever high or low level is present will show up as part of your overall estrogen level. Another factor that can influence the blood test is the form of estrogen that you take. Different forms are absorbed at a different rate.

So how do you utilize blood tests and interpret them accurately?

In my practice, I find it convenient for patients to come in for a blood draw two or three hours after their morning dosage: for capsule users, two hours after; for users of sublingual drops or gel, three hours after. This gives me a peak blood-level reading. This level may be two or three times higher than the average amount circulating in the body later in the day.

Show the chart on page 76 to your physician. A doctor not familiar with using natural estrogen might be alarmed by the high level and discourage you from using the preparation.

If an afternoon blood draw is more convenient, you should do it six to eight hours after taking the estrogen, regardless of the form you use. By then the level should have come down from its earlier peak and fallen into an average range. If your physician is not familiar with natural hormones, you should probably do the afternoon blood draw, or a draw first thing in the morning after a late-night use.

What if your blood test level appears too low to your physician based on the six- or eight-hour blood draw after taking estrogen? If you have no subjective sign of estrogen deficiency you generally don't need to increase your estrogen level. You may want to repeat the test at the peak hormone level two or three hours after taking it.

I consider a reading of more than 500 to 600 pg/ml after two or three hours, or more than 350 after eight hours, to be too high. Usually, you will know if you are taking too much.

If you experience subjective relief from signs of estrogen deficiency and no signs of excess, then you are probably taking an optimum amount. The blood test is really an unsatisfactory tool to obtain the kind of information we want to know: how the estrogen is working and doing its job *inside* the cells. This is where hormones have their impact, and not in the peripheral blood supply that is drawn from your arm. *How you feel—and if you have symptoms or not— provides the best feedback for what is going on in the cells.*

Never forget the individuality factor and how you personally feel. The estrogen type-two woman (tall, slim, and small-breasted) may need only a fifth

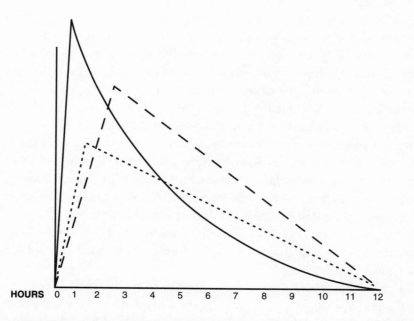

HOURS 0 1 2 3 4 5 6 7 8 9 10 11 12

ESTROGEN BLOOD LEVEL AFTER TAKING SUBLINGUAL DROPS, CAPSULES, GEL

———— Sublingual drops cause the quickest and highest rise in blood level. Estrogen peaks in 1/2 hour to 45 minutes. The decline of blood level with drops is steeper and earlier than other forms.

- - - - - - - Capsules peak earlier than gel and do not drop as steeply as other forms.

— — — Gel creates an estrogen peak after 3 hours, then falls gradually.

of the amount required by the type-one woman (who is smaller, stockier, and full-breasted). If the smaller-framed woman reduces her estrogen intake because her level is relatively high, she may experience many symptoms of deficiency as a result.

Anytime you adjust a dose from either too high or too low, you should repeat the blood test in a month to six weeks to ensure that you are falling in an acceptable range.

If you have been using Premarin or any similar pharmaceutical product previous to switching to a natural estrogen, wait at least eight to twelve weeks before doing a blood test. The equine hormones can distort the accuracy of a blood test. You want them out of your body before you do the test.

Another available test was developed in Europe and analyzes urine over a twenty-four hour period. But it calls for carrying around a specimen container all day. Most women don't want the bother. Moreover, I haven't found this procedure any more useful than the blood test in helping to adjust a patient's individual dosage.

A new test becoming popular involves measuring saliva. I will talk about it more in the progesterone section. But I don't regard it as a practical tool to help adjust dosage.

SHBG Backup

As a safeguard against possible lab errors with the blood hormone test, I check the level of the sex hormone–binding globulin. Remember that the SHBG level goes up when your estrogen level goes up.

If you use the gel, and the SHBG level is high (over 90 nmol/l) and it was lower previously, then the estrogen level is probably too high. Try to decrease the amount. If you accomplish this without developing any signs of deficiency, this means you were indeed taking too much. If the decrease of estrogen produces signs of deficiency, follow your feelings and raise the level to where it was before.

If you previously used any type of a pill and you switch to a natural gel, you should see a decrease of SHBG within two months. If it doesn't decrease by at least 20 percent, you may be taking too much gel. Reduce the amount.

If you start with Tri-Est capsules or drops and hadn't been taking a pharmaceutical estrogen before, your SHBG level should not be over 90 nmol/l. If it is more than 100, switch to the gel. If your level has increased by less than 20 percent from the initial baseline SHBG test, you may not be taking enough estrogen. Increase your dosage.

In general, you don't want to see a SHBG level over 100. If it is over 100 and you are taking capsules or drops, switch to the gel. If it is over 100 and you are using gel, then use less.

Pelvic Ultrasound and Beyond

The role of pelvic ultrasound in hormonal replacement therapy is to measure the thickness of the endometrium, the lining of the uterus. Many of you are in a situation of estrogen dominance, with little or no counterbalancing progesterone. The unopposed estrogen can promote an increase in the thickness of the lining, and could lead to bleeding, polyps, or a precancerous condition.

Ultrasound is a simple office test. It should be performed on a yearly basis, before starting on a hormone program, three months after beginning a program, and at any sign of bleeding. It is good preventive medicine. Any irregularity should be brought to the attention of a gynecologist.

* * *

This may all sound complicated. But it really isn't. Since I am not seeing you in my office, I can't deal with your individual situation. That's why in this book I am covering the most common contingencies I encounter among my patients.

You and your physician simply need to address your own situation—whether you are starting from scratch with natural hormones or have previously taken pharmaceutical products. The monitoring procedures I have described are designed to serve as safeguards to ensure your well-being and detect any unhealthy developments.

9

Natural Estrogen Replacement for Perimenopause

Defining Perimenopause

Perimenopause means "around menopause." Specifically, it refers to the transition from "normality" to menopause, which can occur roughly between forty and fifty-five.

For many women, the transition is a bumpy ride of menstrual irregularity, changes in the amount of bleeding, and unpredictable intervals between periods. Often the signs of perimenopause are confused with intense symptoms of PMS. There is a significant difference between the two. Most of the time, PMS relates to progesterone deficiency. The major symptoms of perimenopause are caused by estrogen deficiency.

Throughout your reproductive years, a week after you ovulate, your body assesses whether you are pregnant. If you are not, your estrogen and progesterone levels drop, leading to the onset of menses. During perimenopause, this drop is steeper and faster.

In addition, many perimenopausal women have erratic pendulum swings of estrogen, ranging from Mount Everest highs to Dead Sea lows.

Laboratory Tests to Confirm Perimenopause

A reading of high FSH (over 15 miu/ml), based on a blood draw during menses, is the major medical criterion defining perimenopause. At the same time, the estrogen blood level may be low, average, or high. Low or average levels, even though within normal limits, could be accompanied by signs of estrogen deficiency. Keep in mind that estrogen starts to decline from about age thirty. Whatever the level is now, it is usually lower than before. However, some women in perimenopause experience a higher level.

Four Groups of Perimenopausal Women

Over the years I have found that perimenopausal women fit into four general categories:

1. Those with intermittent fluctuations.
2. Those with symptoms of gradual estrogen decline most of the time
3. A small percentage who have no symptoms at all.
4. Another group with estrogen excess until a few months before menopause.

Who Should Take Natural Estrogen Replacement?

The answer is simple: *anyone who has signs of estrogen deficiency.* The earlier you intervene the more readily you can prevent symptoms and prolong your inner and outer youthfulness.

If and when you take hormones is clearly a personal decision. You can wait until menopause develops or you can take action as soon as your body signals a deficiency.

If you opt to balance your estrogen now in perimenopause, you should definitely think about balancing progesterone afterward. See chapter 15 on how to balance progesterone.

Unfortunately, increasing numbers of perimenopausal women are prescribed birth control pills. In my opinion, they would be far better served with both natural estrogen and progesterone.

Natural Estrogen for Deficiency Symptoms Due to Intermittent Fluctuations

Sublingual drops (Tri-Est 0.625 milligrams per drop). For mild symptoms, such as the onset of mental fogginess or minor hot flashes, use one to three drops twice daily. Take the drops for as long as you have symptoms. Sometimes you may only need to use them a few days during the cycle.

For more severe symptoms, take three to five drops twice daily. Drops are the most effective and convenient form of estrogen for dealing with typical fluctuations that appear suddenly and without warning. Convenience is the main reason why I recommend drops here. You can carry them with you at all times.

Refer to chapter 7 for details on how to use the sublingual drops.

Natural Estrogen if You Have Symptoms Most of the Time

By perimenopause, about 70 percent of women have lost a third of the estrogen production they had in their midtwenties. Often they trudge to their physician, complaining of symptoms related to estrogen deficiency. The doctor does a blood test to determine the estrogen level. Typically, the reading falls within a huge "normal" range between 50 and 250 pg/ml.

The "normal" reading doesn't mean much if you have symptoms and your level of estrogen is fluctuating daily. I would not trust the blood test here, unless it shows you are at an extreme end. The combination of "normal" and symptoms of deficiency puts you smack in that large group of perimenopausal women who have lost a sizable amount of their estrogen production.

JENNIFER'S STORY

Jennifer, a forty-three-year-old homemaker, was a typical example. She hadn't been sleeping well. From time to time she would wake up and notice she was a little wet from perspiration. She had always prided herself on having a sharp memory, but now she was struggling to remember names and phone numbers. She felt her eyes becoming drier. Her sexual desire had decreased, and she noticed more vaginal friction during intercourse.

I didn't need to test her estrogen level to know what was going on. But she wanted to know. Sure enough, the test for E2 showed her estrogen was in the "normal range."

These symptoms are a clear message from your body. "Fill me up again," it's saying. "My estrogen level is down." Indeed, replacing the lost estrogen will restore what's missing and revive the ebbing signs of youthfulness.

If you identify with all or a few of these symptoms, despite a "normal" range reading, tell your physician that you are experiencing classic signs of estrogen deficiency. Say that you now want to eliminate those symptoms and gain physical, mental, and emotional benefits by increasing your estrogen level. Keep in mind, however, that you do not ever increase your estrogen without taking natural progesterone to balance the estrogen.

I definitely prefer that women replace the estrogen they are losing, rather than taking birth control pills, sleeping pills, antidepressants, and tranquilizers.

In Jennifer's case, I recommended she take 0.625 milligram Tri-Est sublingual drops (one drop equal to 0.625 milligrams of estrogen) intermittently whenever she experienced signs of deficiency. She adjusted the dosage each month because of estrogen fluctuations. In addition, she used progesterone cream (one gram of the 10 percent strength cream twice a day from day fifteen to twenty-eight of her cycle). This program worked well for her. Nearly all her symptoms disappeared.

A note to physicians. If your patient complains of typical signs of low estrogen despite a "normal" range blood test, believe her. She clearly has low enough estrogen—*in her individual situation*—to cause symptoms.

Guidelines for Starting Estrogen if You Have Symptoms Most of the Time

Gel, sublingual drops, or capsules. Follow the same directions as for onset menopause in chapter 8. Often, however, you will need a somewhat smaller amount.

Natural Estrogen for Premenstrual/Menstrual Migraines and Headaches

Think estrogen instead of Tylenol, Advil, or more potent painkillers if you begin experiencing migraines in your forties and early fifties. A great majority of women who develop migraines can significantly benefit from proper estrogen supplementation.

The decline and dramatic fluctuations of estrogen often provide the sparks that set off severe headaches and migraines. In some women this happens throughout the cycle. But physiologically, it is the rapid and steep drop of estrogen a week or so before menstruation and the low level that continues during the period that has the biggest impact. In my experience, the steeper the drop the more dramatic are the symptoms.

The pain is often excruciating and totally disabling for days every month. This is a significant health issue. For many women, their well-being and ability to function normally is severely affected.

Anytime I give estrogen premenstrually, I always add progesterone. I find that some of the premenstrual headaches and migraines can be slightly decreased, but rarely totally relieved, by progesterone alone.

Guidelines for Starting Estrogen for Premenstrual/ Menstrual Migraines

Gel or sublingual drops. Take between ½ to 1½ grams of the basic Tri-Est gel two to four times daily, or two to four drops two to four times a day of the Tri-Est 0.625 drops.

Many of my patients obtain significant relief from the gel or drops. I recommend keeping the hormone handy or in your purse, especially around the time that you tend to get the migraine. If you feel a migraine or headache coming on, immediately take a gram (one-quarter of a teaspoon) of the gel or three drops. Repeat this at least three times for a few days thereafter.

I have found that you can often prevent the migraine or headache by using the following strategies:

- **For migraines during your period only:** Use the sublingual drops or gel two days before menstruation. Stop when your period ends.
- **For migraines before your period:** Use the drops or gel two days prior to the usual onset of symptoms. Continue for the first three days of the period even if the pain is gone. Then stop.
- **For migraines before and during the period:** Use the drops or gel two days earlier than the usual onset of symptoms. Stop at the end of the period.
- **For migraines throughout the cycle:** You may need continual estrogen replacement. If replacement doesn't help in this situation, the migraines are probably not related to estrogen.
- **Using the estrogen patch:** While most women respond to the gel and drops, a few do better with the estrogen patch. The patch I recommend is

Vivelle-Dot, at 0.1 milligram strength. The patch blunts the steep hormonal drop by delivering a steady supply of estradiol.

Follow the strategies above for drops and gel. Change the patch every three days, and not every three and a half days, as the label directs. The reason for this is that the potency of the patch lessens during the last twelve hours.

The patch, as we have seen, contains only one of the estrogen compounds—estradiol (E2). This is an aggressive estrogen, and I prefer for a woman not to continue on estradiol exclusively. I try to discontinue the patch and switch patients to the Tri-Est gel or drops as soon as possible. These formulas contain estriol (E3), which counterbalances the stronger estrogen. Some women who use the patch do not obtain a high enough estrogen boost and also need intermittent use of the gel or drops as well.

Monitoring Your Intake

Do the Estrogen Quick Check twice a day. I describe how to do it in the previous chapter. Use the Quick Check for as long as you feel your estrogen level is fluctuating and you need to change your dosages. Skip it once you feel your level has stabilized and you are not readjusting frequently.

If you suffer from headaches or migraines, the prevention or relief of pain will serve as your dosage guide. Sometimes you may have to use more estrogen than usual to achieve your goal. Once symptoms are gone or tolerable, you may want to try to slowly lower your dosage throughout the day.

Monitoring Your Intake with Your Physician

Women with symptoms of low estrogen. Have an estrogen blood test done during the eighteenth to twenty-first day of your cycle, six to eight hours after taking estrogen. I recommend the test to make sure that you are not among the few women who take too much estrogen yet do not show signs of excess.

Women with menstrual or premenstrual headaches/migraines. My concern is that you don't take too much natural estrogen in order to prevent the onset of severe pain.

Have an estrogen blood test during the eighteenth to twenty-first day of your cycle, when you are not taking any extra estrogen. Then retest while you are taking the estrogen during your headache period. Have the blood drawn six to eight hours after your morning estrogen intake. If the level of the estrogen is higher than the first reading, try to decrease your dosage.

What If You Have Symptoms of Too Much Estrogen?

An overproduction of estrogen by your ovaries can occur when the body's hormonal regulatory mechanisms are not functioning correctly. This happens frequently during perimenopause. As a result, you may experience water retention and breast enlargement, or become antsy and uptight.

Parallel to the unpredictable gyrations of estrogen, the level of progesterone declines rapidly during perimenopause. Progesterone is the great hormonal harmonizer and protector. It balances estrogen. With the decline of progesterone, we see a rising influence of "unopposed" estrogen and an increase in the incidence of fibroids, polyps, endometriosis, adenomyosis, irregular bleeding, and hysterectomies. This hormonal environment can also promote the development of a precancerous condition in the uterus and theoretically reduce breast protection.

My goal with patients is to try to reduce the risks associated with a high level of estrogen.

Two laboratory tests can help confirm the existence of excess estrogen. The first is a blood test for estradiol (E2) taken between five to nine days before menses. A reading over 250 pg/ml indicates excess estrogen. I have seen women with levels over 1,000 pg/ml produced by their own bodies.

At the same time, test the level for the sex hormone–binding globulin. A reading of over 90 nmol/l indicates excess estrogen. Remember that when the level of estrogen goes up, SHBG rises with it. Estrogen, whether you produce it in your body or take it as part of a hormone replacement program, can raise SHBG.

The numbers I have used here are for "average" patients. Some women have relatively low estrogen until they enter perimenopause and then they, too, experience the upward fluctuations of estrogen. On the blood test, they will probably have a much lower E2 value than "average," but could still have symptoms of excess estrogen.

What to Do in Case of Subjective and Laboratory Evidence of Excess Estrogen

Follow the guidelines below for as long as you experience symptoms.

1. *Take natural progesterone.* Ask your physician for a prescription. This is your primary weapon and often may be all you need to do.

2. *Take a soy phytoestrogen (isoflavone) supplement.* These products are available in health food stores. Refer to the section on estrogen substitutes at the end of chapter 7. Take 100 to 200 milligrams of isoflavones daily.

3. Use natural agents to eliminate excess estrogen. Once molecules of estrogen have performed their cellular mission, they are carried to the liver and *deactivated.* From there they are transported to the gastrointestinal tract for eventual excretion. However, an enzyme in the intestines called beta-glucuronidase *reactivates* some of the estrogen, allowing it to be reabsorbed back into the bloodstream. This recycling process produces about 30 percent of the available estrogen in your body. We can interfere with the recycling operation, and thus reduce the total estrogen load, by taking two supplements, both of which are available at health food stores.

- **Fiber.** Use any good fiber supplement except the water-soluble type. Follow label instructions. Studies have shown that fiber can bind up to 30 percent of the excess estrogen in the intestinal tract.
- **Calcium d-glucarate (CDG).** Take 400 milligrams twice daily with meals. This substance blocks beta-glucuronidase activity and prevents the recycling of the outward-bound estrogen. CDG is made in small quantities by the body. It is also found naturally in many fruits and vegetables.

4. Fortify your liver. The strategy is to improve the liver's ability to perform its original deactivation of estrogen. You can accomplish this by giving optimum nutritional support to the liver and reducing its exposure to liver toxic substances, such as alcohol.

The key liver supplements I recommend to patients are:

- Inositol and choline (B complex vitamins), 100 milligrams each daily.
- The amino acids methionine, 100 milligrams daily, and N-acetyl cysteine, 500 milligrams twice daily.
- Alpha lipoic acid (an antioxidant), 500 milligrams twice daily.

Try to reduce the use of alcohol and Tylenol, which have harmful effects on the liver. Eat wholesome food, and try to avoid food with chemical additives.

5. Indole-3 carbinole. Take 400 milligrams daily of this remarkably protective supplement. Indole is found naturally in broccoli, cabbage, and other *Brassica* family vegetables. The supplement can help reduce the transformation of estrogen into precancerous metabolites.

EILEEN'S STORY—THE TRIBULATIONS OF PERIMENOPAUSE

Eileen was forty-four years old when I first saw her. This mother of three was not what I would call typically perimenopausal, but she had so many of the problems related to perimenopause that I want to share her story with you.

On her first appointment, Eileen told me that during the previous two years she was having more difficulty falling asleep. Sometimes she would wake up in sweat during the middle of the night.

She complained of fuzzy thinking and becoming increasingly emotional. She would cry easily, and feel anxious and depressed before her period. She said her breasts were not as full as they used to be. She was retaining water.

"In the beginning I was uncomfortable before and during my period," she told me when I asked for more details. "Then all these things began happening erratically throughout my whole cycle. Lately, I feel they are all getting worse. And now I have started to develop bad migraines before my period."

Eileen said she felt the best after her period and until ovulation. This obviously meant that her body produced the most estrogen at this time.

If I had seen her two years before I would have started her on small amounts of estrogen four or five days before her period and continuing throughout the period. I would have added progesterone from day fifteen to twenty-eight.

If I had seen her the year before I would have recommended she now take estrogen throughout the cycle and adjust her doses as needed.

But her symptoms had now progressed. They were broader, more intense, and of longer duration. She was now having difficulty sleeping during the whole month. She was often waking up in the morning with a foggy mind and little enthusiasm for the day's activities. Her moods were unpredictable. One day she would feel great. The next day she would be depressed. Her energy fluctuated dramatically. And now, to make things worse, she was having migraines.

Endocrine workups revealed relatively low E2 (40 pg/ml) and SHBG (50 nmol/l), and a high FSH (over 15 miu/ml) at the beginning of her cycle. Her blood level of progesterone on day twenty-one was 7 ng/ml.

Analyzing her situation, the following was clear:

Eileen's problems began with plunging estrogen prior to her period along with an overall decline of progesterone. These two developments were triggering premenstrual symptoms. The depression, night sweats, difficulty falling asleep, and premenstrual migraines were due to estrogen deficiency. The anxiety, water retention, tendency to cry, as well as some breast tenderness, were related mostly to progesterone.

I recommended Tri-Est sublingual drops daily throughout the month and adjusting the dosage as needed. I asked her to increase the amount and frequency for a few days before her period and continuing for a few days after it ended to prevent the migraines. This program worked well for almost a year. She now returned to see me and complained of water retention, breast tenderness, and feeling edgy and uptight throughout the whole cycle.

When such symptoms appear during the entire month, and not just premenstrually, or when it appears with women who are menopausal and don't have cycles, the cause is usually estrogen excess.

Sometimes the symptoms can represent progesterone deficiency, but here in Eileen's case, the blood tests incriminated estrogen. A blood workup revealed a high level of both estrogen and SHBG. A pelvic ultrasound showed the presence of a simple ovarian cyst.

As I said at the beginning of the chapter, a woman in perimenopause may go through wild swings of estrogen, from very low to very high. Here, the estrogen level had soared. The rise was further compounded by the cyst, which caused more estrogen to be produced. I stopped her estrogen replacement.

Three months later when I saw Eileen again, the estrogen level had come back down. Six months later, she was thrown into a nearly complete menopausal state and needed to resume estrogen replacement. Such scenarios, which involve a significant rise in estrogen preceding a major drop into menopause, are not uncommon.

Eileen's predicament contains hormonal subplots that often take place at this stage of a woman's life. Many of you will experience some of the symptoms associated with these changes. Some of you will experience all of them. But everyone can significantly reduce them by using natural hormones.

10

Natural Estrogen Replacement for Younger Women

WHAT'S IN THIS CHAPTER

- Who should take natural estrogen?
- If you have infrequent or no periods
- If you are tall, thin, and flat-chested with signs of estrogen deficiency
- Monitoring your progress with your physician
- The effect of the birth control pill on your estrogen
- Amber's story: problems with the pill

Who Should Take Natural Estrogen?

To say that hormones are raging in a young woman is meaningless. The issue is whether these hormones are crying for balance.

It is equally meaningless to say that just because a woman is young she doesn't need estrogen. There are individuals who require it. This chapter focuses on those particular women.

If You Have Infrequent or No Periods

Young women prone to have infrequent periods, or no periods at all, are individuals whose hormonal systems are not yet fully developed, or who are underweight, anorectic, or overexercising. Their estrogen blood levels range from low to the extremely low values seen in menopause.

Ask your physician to test your estrogen, FSH, and SHBG levels.

You are probably producing a normal amount of estrogen if you have no signs of deficiency and your estradiol (E2) reading is between 50 and 250 pg/ml, your FSH under 7 miu/ml, and your sex hormone–binding globulin level higher than 50 nmol/l.

The fact that you are not ovulating means your body is not producing progesterone. As a result, you have estrogen dominance. Theoretically, this could threaten your long-term health. The solution is to take natural progesterone, which I will discuss in chapter 16.

Within this category are women who produce less estrogen than they need. Their estradiol value is always in a menopausal range, that is, less than 50 picograms, sometimes lower than 20, or even below the level that the laboratory can measure. Unlike menopause, the FSH level is depressed or normal, but never high (over 10 miu/ml). FSH, you will remember, is the hormone produced by the pituitary gland that tells your ovaries to make more estrogen. The SHBG level is low, nearly always under 50 nmol/l.

In these cases, the hypothalamus, the brain center that governs overall hormone activity in the body, is not functioning correctly. This can be due to immaturity of the system and lack of fatty tissue in the body. You can have all the physical signs, and many of the subjective signs, of estrogen deficiency that are found in menopause. And indeed you don't have enough estrogen.

You should not be treated, as many women are in this situation, with birth control pills. The pill does not give your system a chance to normalize. The pill delivers chemicalized hormones that are totally foreign to the body, further suppressing an already suppressed and out-of-balance system. The exquisite hormonal choreography conducted by your brain center is compromised. The brain gets the message that you have enough hormones, so it doesn't ask the body to make more. The pill is a fundamental mistake in this situation, a daily insult to your body and your evolution.

You should only take natural hormonal replacement. This gives the body a greater opportunity to achieve balance on its own.

If you don't address the problem with natural hormones, you are left with all the signs of menopause and accelerated aging. You will lose bone. You will lose cardiovascular protection. You will lose skin elasticity.

If you are in this particular group, and not producing adequate estrogen, should you supplement yourself in such a way to restore your period? For many individuals, menstruation is a primordial rite associated with womanhood. This is a personal decision. Healthwise, there is no advantage to restoring the period. But if you choose to have it, be sure to take progesterone two weeks out of every month. See chapter 16 for the guidelines.

Taking estrogen and progesterone on a daily basis provides long-term protection for the health of the breasts, uterus, and probably the ovaries as well. This mimics the ideal protective mode of the body during pregnancy, when hormonal levels are high.

How Much—and in What Form—Should You Take?

This group of women experiences few or minor estrogen fluctuations. To replace estrogen, follow the guidelines for women in mid-menopause.

Monitoring Your Intake

Do the Estrogen Quick Test (see page 72).

Once you are on a replacement program, be alert to the possibility that your ovaries can start producing estrogen at any time. It is hard to predict when that will happen. Each situation is individual.

For some very young women, it might take years for the system to mature enough before an adequate level is produced. For a woman with anorexia, it could happen when she starts eating normally and gains weight. For women who stop taking the birth control pill, it could happen once the body recovers from the hormonal suppression caused by the pill.

You will know your body is making estrogen if you begin developing signs of too much estrogen (see p. 29). The signs are your cue to reduce intake. If the signs of excess estrogen continue, stop the hormone supplement. There's no need to resume it as long as you are comfortable and feel the benefits of your own estrogen.

Monitoring Your Progress with Your Physician

Check your E2 and SHBG blood levels six to eight hours after taking estrogen. You should see an E2 level under 250 pg/ml and a sex hormone–binding globulin level around 80 nmol/l. If the values are higher, reduce your dosage.

If You Are Tall, Thin, and Flat-chested with Signs of Estrogen Deficiency

Your physical structure tells you that only a small amount of estrogen is present in the body. This explains your height. There was not enough estrogen available to close bone formation and arrest upward growth. This explains why your breasts may be smaller. There was not enough estrogen available to fully potentiate the estrogen-sensitive breast tissue.

On natural estrogen replacement, many women of this body type suddenly thrive. That's because the missing ingredient has been restored and now generates a better level of function.

Some women may not be helped. I understand from this that their bodies are competent to operate on a lesser quantity of estrogen. They function perfectly well—mentally, emotionally, and physically—on less.

However, if signs of low estrogen are present then estrogen replacement is always beneficial. To recognize the signs refer to the beginning of chapter 5. Many times there are no signs because of the body's adaptation to low estrogen.

I look for additional indicators, such as a *persistent subtle depression* that seems to take away much of the joy of life. The person tends to be apathetic, with no anxiety or emotional ups and downs. Such women may feel better on the birth control pill and when they are pregnant. That's because the body is responding positively to getting more than the accustomed low level of estrogen. This response indicates that proper estrogen replacement can be very beneficial.

How Much—and in What Form—Should You Take?

Any form of estrogen—capsules, drops, or gel—will be helpful. The higher doses below should be used for a week before, and during, menstruation. This provides extra estrogen when the ovaries naturally produce less.

Use the lower doses in the second and third week of the cycle when production is higher. You can try to add more at any time if you obtain additional benefits. Always be sure to counterbalance any additional estrogen with extra progesterone (see chapter 16).

Guidelines for Starting

Sublingual drops. (Tri-Est 0.625-milligram strength per drop) One or two drops twice a day.

Gel. (the basic Tri-Est combination of 0.25 milligrams of estrone, 0.75 milligrams of estradiol, and 2.5 milligrams of estriol in each gram of gel): ¼ to ½ gram twice a day.

Capsules. (Tri-Est 0.625-milligram strength per capsule): One or two capsules twice a day.

Monitoring Your Intake

Do the Estrogen Quick Check on p. 72. It will help you determine if you are taking too much.

Monitoring Your Progress with Your Physician

Obtain an E2 blood test during your period, six to eight hours after taking estrogen. You don't want to see a level exceeding 200 pg/ml. Most women in this category cannot tolerate higher doses without developing the side effects of excess estrogen.

The Effect of the Birth Control Pill on Your Estrogen

Many of my patients ask my opinion about using the birth control pill. This is a difficult question. On the one hand, most women are understandably reluctant to bring a dozen children into the world. On the other hand, the birth control pill is not perfect.

The pill contains patented chemicalized estrogen substitutes that are totally different from the estrogen in your body, along with a chemicalized progesterone substitute called progestin that is derived from male testosterone.

The pill suppresses ovulation. This occurs through the action of the pill's estrogen drug. This substance is not quickly metabolized by the liver, as is your own natural hormone. It remains in the body at a high level and thus exerts a suppressive effect on the ovaries.

Putting the basic issue of birth control aside, let's examine the pros and cons of the pill in relation to estrogen.

The upside. The pill protects against uterine and ovarian cancer, preserves fertility, and reduces the incidence of endometriosis.

The downside. Most of the time the estrogen content of the standard pill increases the sex hormone–binding globulin. As I have said earlier, any form of oral estrogen affects SHBG. When the SHBG level goes up, the benefits of important antiaging hormones are reduced. These hormones, which circulate in the body, become increasingly bound up and prevented from carrying out their specific hormonal duties. The benefits from thyroid hormone, human growth hormone, and testosterone are all decreased.

A second problem is that the pill contains only aggressive estrogen. There is no trace of the estriol (E3) fraction of estrogen, which provides many protective and balancing benefits. This might in part explain the increase in breast cancer among women who took the pill when they were younger.

When my patients tell me they want to start the pill, I offer them a number of guidelines:

1. Always keep your liver in tip-top shape. Follow the liver fortifying program I described in the previous chapter. This will help your liver process any excess estrogen in your body.

2. Prior to starting the pill, measure the estradiol (E2) and SHBG levels on day twenty-one of the cycle in order to determine your estrogen status. It is useful to have these baseline measurements on hand as a comparison to help determine later if the estrogen content in the pill is too high or too low for you. If you experience signs of excess estrogen, such as breast enlargement, water retention, or irritability, ask your physician to give you a pill with less estrogen. Signs of low estrogen mean the pill doesn't have enough of the hormone for you. Ask your physician for a pill with more estrogen. Doctors today are prescribing pills with a much lower estrogen level than before. As a result we tend to see more women showing signs of deficiency.

3. Many side effects from the pill are caused by its progestin contents. I will talk much more about that in chapter 12. That will give you a good idea of what you are swallowing.

4. Women are bombarded these days with advertisements pushing the pill as a solution to acne problems. Here's how the pill may help your acne: the pill increases the level of SHBG, which binds some of the testosterone a woman produces in her body. If the acne is related to an overproduction of testosterone, as it often is, then the pill may help you. It's also very possible that you may not benefit. That's because most of the progestin used in the pill is produced from chemicalized testosterone. Thus, you may develop symptoms of excess testosterone, and they *include* acne. I have found many times that acne relief depends totally on the right pill for the right person.

5. I never prescribe the pill to a patient in order to regulate her period. Unfortunately, as I have said before, this is being done frequently and can cause much hormonal chaos. Women need to be regulated only with what their body is missing—the natural estrogen or progesterone that is identical to the hormones produced by their own body.

AMBER'S STORY: PROBLEMS FROM THE PILL

Amber was seventeen years old, five foot six, 125 pounds, with small breasts. She had her first period at the age of fifteen and then menstruated irregularly. Another physician placed her on the birth control pill.

She came to see me complaining of multiple symptoms. She had severe breast tenderness, water retention, decreased sex drive, fatigue in the morning, and cold extremities. She noticed that she hardly ever perspired with exertion. She was upset at having gained twenty pounds since starting the birth control pill.

Amber was like many young women. She didn't produce a great deal of estrogen. That's why she was relatively tall, her breasts small, and why she began menstruating later than most of her girlfriends.

Her endocrine system had been very slow to mature. She never ovulated. And that's why her periods were irregular. Her estrogen level, even though low, was sufficient for her. She didn't have any signs of estrogen deficiency.

By putting her on the pill, she was introduced to a higher level of estrogen than her body needed. This was a physiological mistake. Her immature system was further suppressed. Its opportunity to wake up and bloom was inhibited.

The signs of excess estrogen caused by the pill were breast tenderness and water retention. The pill increased her SHBG level and thus decreased the availability of other hormones inside the body, such as her own ovarian testosterone. One effect of this was a lowered sex drive.

The higher SHBG also decreased the availability of thyroid hormone, which caused weight gain, fatigue, coldness in the hands and feet, and interfered with her ability to sweat. These were indications to me of thyroid deficiency caused by the pill.

Amber didn't need the pill. *She needed progesterone.*

While her own estrogen production was very low, without progesterone to balance it, even this low level was enough to create a situation of estrogen dominance. Here we take a very young woman who already has a small degree of estrogen dominance two weeks out of every month and we increase the dominance further with the pill!

I stopped the pill. I started her on progesterone two weeks out of the month in order to restore her period, which was very essential for her.

All her symptoms disappeared.

Ideally, I would have liked her to take progesterone daily throughout the month, not just for two weeks to create a regular period. I would also have added estriol (E3) to create a hormonal environment present during the normal cycle. This would give her the best long-term protection from breast, uterine, and ovarian cancer.

Two years later, Amber developed estrogen deficiency. Why? She had embarked on a vigorous exercise program in order to participate in marathon runs. With this development, she stopped having her period, despite the fact that she was taking progesterone two weeks out of the month. Blood work demonstrated low E2 and SHBG.

Interpretation: the heavy exercise had decreased her body fat, which resulted in her body producing even less estrogen than it did before. The decrease was enough now to create symptoms of deficiency. Now, she needed a complete daily replacement with estrogen.

Three years later, Amber was treated for infertility with hormonal injections. She had a successful twin pregnancy, and seven months after childbirth, she started to have regular periods with good hormonal balance.

The final analysis of Amber's story? We see how women's bodies change and grow with the woman. The role of hormone replacement therapy changes also to suit each woman's current goals.

Additionally, Amber's story also illustrates how childbirth can bring on a more normal hormonal picture, even if the pregnancy has to be induced pharmaceutically.

PART THREE

How to Optimize Your Progesterone Protection

11

ABCs of Progesterone

WHAT'S IN THIS CHAPTER

- Progesterone at a glance
- Benefits of natural progesterone replacement
- Common signs of progesterone deficiency
- The meaning of your progesterone blood level

Progesterone at a Glance

Immediately after a woman ovulates, her ovaries produce progesterone, the hormone that prepares the uterus for the reception and development of the fertilized egg.

Progesterone's name tells its function: *pro* means "for," and *gest* means "gestation." It plays a major role in a woman's ability to conceive and sustain the pregnancy.

In addition to this fundamental role in conception, progesterone provides many major protective functions to the body. Among the most important is its role as the great "hormonal harmonizer." It balances estrogen. Anytime that the estrogen level rises in the body, you want to have progesterone there to offset it. That's why I like to refer to it as the "estrogen shock absorber."

A female has little progesterone until she begins ovulating. For some, this can be as early as ten years of age. For others, it never occurs naturally and needs to be induced through modern medical intervention.

Unlike estrogen, the body never overproduces progesterone. It does, however, manufacture a large amount of the hormone during pregnancy, which serves to promote the development of the fetus.

In a normal twenty-eight-day menstrual cycle, barely any progesterone is

99

produced during the first two weeks. After ovulation, at day fourteen, progesterone kicks in. The level peaks at day twenty-one. If no fertilization takes place, the body pulls the switch on progesterone and the hormone level starts falling. The mechanism is precise. The progesterone phase lasts for two weeks after ovulation.

If the period comes earlier, the body is not producing enough progesterone. If the period does not come at all, it is a typical sign of pregnancy. However, longer intervals or no periods at all are also signs of progesterone deficiency.

I find that women with progesterone deficiency tend to get their first period relatively late. They have a history of infrequent periods with minor bleeding. They often have difficulty becoming pregnant or carrying the pregnancy to term.

In the life cycle, women generally start to produce less progesterone when they reach their early thirties. The slowdown increases after thirty-five, and accelerates dramatically in the forties. Very few women over forty-five produce the quantity of progesterone that they did twenty years earlier. In perimenopause, most of them are deficient in progesterone.

Some women in perimenopause may experience fluctuations that occur in blocks. They may ovulate, for instance, for several months at a time and then stop ovulating for several months. But there are none of the frequent ups and downs that take place on a daily or weekly basis, as with estrogen. For more than 60 percent of women, the decline is persistent.

All women in menopause are progesterone-deficient. They have only a minute amount of progesterone, a level insufficient to carry out the hormone's widespread physiological tasks. One of those critical tasks is to generate new bone tissue. The loss of this function is a major contributing factor to osteoporosis.

This overall reduction in progesterone is earlier, more rapid and persistent than the decline of estrogen. The departure of progesterone from the hormonal stage leaves the body vulnerable to the consequences of estrogen dominance. The loss of hormonal balance is a root cause of many female problems, such as endometriosis, fibroids, polyps, adenomyosis, irregular periods, heavy bleeding, and out-of-control cycles.

Benefits of Natural Progesterone Replacement

In this age of estrogen dominance, I believe that a woman should always consider taking natural progesterone.

I routinely recommend it to patients whenever they take estrogen. I want a woman to have the important balancing and harmonizing effects that progesterone offers. This simple strategy could theoretically decrease the incidence of cancer, prolong the regularity of menstruation, and generate numerous health benefits.

Here's what progesterone can do for you, and what some of my patients have said after using it:

- It protects the breasts, uterus, and probably the ovaries from cancer.
- It acts as a natural diuretic: "I lost five pounds of water."
- It produces a calming, antianxiety effect: "You don't know how good it feels to be in control of my emotions again."
- It decreases PMS and menstrual flow: "Now I am the same women for the whole month."
- It enhances your body's defenses.
- It improves the breakdown of fat into energy.
- It cuts the craving for carbohydrates and sweets: "I don't need my M&M's fix anymore."
- It reduces breast tenderness and pain: "My breasts are mine again."
- It contributes to the formation of new bone tissue.
- It increases HDL, the body's "good cholesterol."

Although I have read reports that progesterone decreases hot flashes and promotes skin and vaginal lubrication, I tend to discount them. I have seen such effects from progesterone only on rare occasions. Estrogen replacement, however, will accomplish this.

Common Signs of Progesterone Deficiency

- Amenorrhea—no period at all. There is no ovulation. The ovaries are producing only a bare minimum of progesterone. Frequently, patients tell me, "I just want to have a period."
- Oligomenorrhea—the period comes infrequently, perhaps every few months. This is also a result of minimum progesterone production. "Is such a small flow healthy?" patients want to know.
- Heavy and frequent periods. This situation could be related to tissue buildup in the uterus because of prolonged progesterone deficiency. "I get frightened when I see the large clots," patients often say.
- Spotting a few days before the period. Here, the progesterone level is drop-

ping rapidly and prematurely during the monthly cycle. Patients will tell me they "don't like to use pads for so long."

- PMS. Most PMS symptoms, whether physical or emotional, are progesterone-related. Initially, they may occur for a few days before the period. The more severe the deficiency, the longer they last. They may persist from the time of ovulation until the onset of the period. Many a patient has told me that "for a few days out of the month, I don't like the person I become."
- Cystic breasts. "The cysts in my breasts scare me."
- Painful breasts. "When my husband hugs me I have a lot of pain."
- Breasts with lumps. "When I feel the lumps my heart stops."
- Most cases of endometriosis, adenomyosis, and fibroids. "I will take anything to get rid of this."
- Anxiety, irritability, and nervousness. Difficulty sleeping and relaxing. "I have become a nervous wreck."
- Water retention. "I can't fit into my shoes."

The Meaning of Your Progesterone Blood Level

Interpreting progesterone and estrogen blood levels are two different propositions. With estrogen, one woman with a blood level of 50 pg/ml might have no symptoms of deficiency while a second woman with a much higher level of 200 pg/ml could indeed have some deficiency symptoms. This wide range of individuality doesn't allow us to use a blood-level reading as a precise instrument for determining optimum dosage in an estrogen replacement program. We rely primarily on how a woman feels, as long as the blood level is within an acceptable range.

There is significantly less variability with progesterone. We also go by how a woman feels, but here we use the blood test reading to help us reach an *optimum zone* where we like to see the progesterone level. Most women can adjust their intake of progesterone to reach that target zone. Others cannot. They will develop signs of excess.

At most laboratories, the optimum zone ranges between 15 to 25 ng/ml. In the labs that I use, the zone is 18 to 20.

I attempt to elevate my patients to this level, without incurring any of the side effects, so they achieve the systemic benefits of progesterone. In chapter 13 I will discuss the many benefits associated with progesterone as well as the possible signs of excess that some women may develop.

Your ability to achieve an optimum level with maximum benefits depends a great deal on the form of progesterone you take. I will go into detail about that as well in chapter 13.

Usually the progesterone range of normal in most labs is between 5 and 25 ng/ml. A level higher than 5 tells us one critical fact—that a woman is ovulating.

Progesterone should be tested a week before the period (usually between day nineteen and twenty-one), when the hormone is at its normal peak level in a twenty-eight-day cycle.

12

Progesterone and Progestins
Two Million Years of Difference

About Progestins

Progestins, or progestogens, as they are sometimes called, are patented, chemicalized, progesterone substitutes. They are not the same as the progesterone your body produces. Unfortunately, nobody tells you otherwise. You hear the word *progestin* and you think they are talking about progesterone.

These substances have some of the actions of the natural progesterone your body makes but *a lot of disturbing side effects as well.*

There are two basic types of progestins. The best known, and most widely used, includes Provera (medroxyprogesterone acetate), and its generic look-alikes. They are derived from a synthetic replica of your own progesterone and then altered chemically.

The other type, derived from a synthetic replica of testosterone, is altered chemically and combined with chemicalized estrogen in birth control pills.

The role of progestins in contraceptives is to generate a thick mucus in the cervix that blocks the sperm from reaching the ovum.

Progestins were added to estrogen replacement therapy when it was established that unopposed estrogen could cause endometrial overgrowth and increase the risk of uterine cancer. Progestins were found to prevent the overgrowth of endometrial tissue and thus lower the risk of this type of cancer.

I don't know if it is human arrogance at work, or the profit motive, but I never understood why researchers wouldn't simply open their physiology books and see how nature prevents this risky imbalance in the first place. Nature prevents it effectively with progesterone, the natural female hormone that balances estrogen. This is the intelligence of a woman's body at work.

Provera (medroxyprogesterone acetate) and its copies indeed help prevent uterine cancer, which, by the way, is a relatively benign form of cancer. But beyond this, the similarity between progestins and progesterone starts to disintegrate. *The fact is that progestins are drugs with side effects.*

The Heart Connection

Before natural progesterone was so widely available I heard many women complain of chest pains after they started taking Provera, even when they used it for a relatively short period of time to balance their periods. Often other physicians had told them they were just nervous or stressed.

Now we know it was not nerves or stress.

Today, growing numbers of cardiologists are openly warning other doctors about Provera. *Specifically, the drug is coronary constrictive. That means it reduces the diameter of the arteries leading to the heart.*

Whenever I mention this issue to cardiologists, they seem to be well aware of the problem.

Several years ago at a medical conference given at Cedars-Sinai Medical Center in Los Angeles, a leading cardiologist commented on the serious side effects of Provera during a lecture. Then, at the end of his talk, he spoke in a hushed voice and suggested to the physicians in attendance not to use Provera. I wondered at the time why he wasn't screaming this warning from the rooftops. And I wonder why the message hasn't yet reached the media and the vast number of women taking Provera.

When men die from heart attacks, as much as 95 percent of their coronary arteries may be clogged. *When women die from heart attacks, only 30 percent have clogged arteries. The main concern with women is not atherosclerosis, narrow-*

ing plaques that form on the inside of the arteries. The major problem is constricted arteries. The blood vessels become squeezed and narrow, choking vital blood flow to the heart muscle. The result of such constriction: sudden-onset heart attacks and severe angina.

Women tend to focus more on the high-profile issue of breast cancer. *Yet heart disease has been the major killer of women for decades.* About 235,000 women die from heart attacks annually in the United States, a figure five times higher than fatalities from breast cancer.

Young men suffer more heart attacks than young women, but women start to close the gap at menopause and eventually have about the same incidence as men, according to the famous Framingham Heart Study. Women under fifty, however, are twice as likely to die from heart attacks as their male peers.

Estrogen is well known for its many protective benefits for the heart. And in younger women, of course, there is a much higher level than in older women. This would help explain in part the age-related increase in heart attacks. We know from studies that estrogen replacement alone may reduce the risk of coronary heart disease in women by up to 50 percent.

Current research shows that estradiol and the standard chemicalized estrogen replacement Premarin have a powerful and positive effect on cardiovascular health and the prevention of heart attacks and strokes. They increase "good" cholesterol and decrease "bad" cholesterol, improve coronary artery dilation and blood flow, and act as an antioxidant, inhibiting the oxidation of the "bad" cholesterol involved in the buildup of unhealthy arterial plaque. These forms of estrogen also protect against insulin irregularities that can lead to diabetes, cardiovascular disease, and increased fat in the abdomen, thighs, and buttocks.

We also know that if you take the commonly prescribed pharmaceutical combinations of estrogen and progestin, the heart-helping benefit of estrogen is lost. The progestin cancels it out and increases the risk.

Two animal experiments reported in 1997 dramatized the potential danger of Provera. Both involved monkeys with ovaries previously removed surgically to simulate menopause.

In one study at the Oregon Regional Primate Research Center, researchers determined that estradiol relaxed the coronary artery and resisted the effect of a chemical known to constrict the artery. When they gave the monkeys natural progesterone there was no loss of estradiol protection. But when Provera was added, the animals experienced arterial spasms so severe that the surprised researchers had to intervene with an antidote.

The addition of Provera, the researchers found, did two things:

1. It canceled the protective effect of estradiol, and
2. It promoted constriction of the coronary arteries to a significant degree beyond that of the artery-constricting chemical alone.

In another experiment at Wake Forest University, researchers fed a special diet to monkeys over a thirty-month period that created atherosclerosis (plaque) in the coronary arteries. The animals were divided into four groups: one was placed on a continual hormonal replacement therapy with the estrogen formulation Premarin alone, a second group on Premarin plus Provera, a third group on Provera alone, and a fourth that received no hormones.

At the end of the study, the monkeys on Premarin had 72 percent less plaque than all the other three groups. The researchers concluded that estrogen "inhibits the initiation and progression of coronary artery atherosclerosis" and that continuously administered progestin "antagonizes" this protective effect.

There are a number of human studies that also point out the negative effect of progestins. At King's College in England, female patients with heart disease were tested for endurance on treadmills. After they were given estrogen for a period of time, they were able to walk longer. However, when Provera was added to the Premarin, they were able to walk less than they had before starting Premarin. The conclusion was that the progestin eliminated the benefit of estrogen and reduced cardiovascular function.

At a 1999 symposium of the American Society for Reproductive Medicine, Janice D. Wagner, Ph.D., of the Wake Forest University School of Medicine, summarized current scientific findings on hormonal replacement and cardiovascular risks. "Accumulating evidence confirms the deleterious effects of medroxyprogesterone (Provera) on estrogen's cardioprotective effects, and provides new and compelling evidence that not all progestogens are alike in this regard," she said.

In her analysis, Wagner noted that Provera undermines the protective benefits related to plaque formation, coronary artery dilation, and cholesterol oxidation, and that it also contributes significantly to insulin resistance.

Other progestogens (progestins), including newly developed products, also reduce the cardiovascular benefits of estrogens to varying degrees.

In plain English, all this means more fat, oxidative damage, heart disease, and diabetes. The findings clearly explain why researchers conclude that hormonal replacement therapy doesn't protect you from cardiovascular disease. The reason is not because of the estrogen component, but because of the negative effect of the progestins.

Wagner pointed out that research indicates natural progesterone protects the endometrium "while preserving the beneficial effects of estrogen on the cardiovascular system." This should come as no surprise. If it had a negative effect, pregnancy would be a serious risk factor for a heart attack. That's the time when the progesterone level rises dramatically. Your own progesterone has no negative effect on the blood vessels that supply your heart.

The incriminating data on Provera is not new. Yet this horrifying drug continues to be widely prescribed to women. Why?

And why aren't women clearly informed about the danger so they can make an educated choice?

The incidence of deadly heart attacks among young women is alarming. Women should ask their physician about potential harm to their cardiovascular health before agreeing to take any progestin.

Currently, the manufacturers of patented, chemicalized hormonal substitutes are spending huge amounts of money on research to come up with progestins that don't have negative effects on the cardiovascular system. They should be required to prove that these new-generation progestins do not close the coronary arteries of women who use them, or have other harmful effects in the body. We shouldn't have to wait twenty years before we find out that they are putting women in the grave.

Emerging research, however, is indicating that the new progestins being developed for the marketplace, such as norgestimate and levonorgestrel, reduce the benefits of estradiol on the oxidation of "bad" cholesterol.

There is, of course, a simple alternative—natural progesterone. A woman does not have to choose between a heart attack and uterine cancer.

The Breast Cancer Connection

One major epidemiological study reported in 1981 that women in their forties with a high level of their own progesterone have one-fifth the rate of breast cancer and one-tenth the rate of other cancers in later life than women with low progesterone. Moreover, there have been a number of other studies reported during the last ten to fifteen years showing how the presence of progesterone enhances the prognosis for women who develop breast cancer.

Progesterone protects the breasts through many mechanisms. Here are some examples:

- It enhances a protective gene system (known as P53). This system slows down another gene system (BCL2) that promotes cancer.

- It "down-regulates" (decreases) survivin, a gene that acts similar to cancer-promoting BCL2.
- It prevents cells from proliferating excessively (dividing faster) in breast and uterine tissue. In one study, researchers found that aggressive estrogen could promote breast cell proliferation by 230 percent, while progesterone, applied as a topical cream to the breasts, decreased the activity by 400 percent.
- It enhances natural killer cells and interleuken-2, two important components of the body's defense system.
- It increases apoptosis, also known as cell "suicide." This process deters cells from mutating into harmful forms due to oxidative and chemical reactions in the body. Estradiol (E2) slows down apoptosis.
- It reduces the ability of breast cancer cells to metastasize.

Do progestins offer similar protection? The research is confusing. In some epidemiological studies on the standard combined drug combination of Premarin and Provera, the inclusion of the progestin appears to increase the risk of breast cancer. One study, in fact, found a disturbing connection between an increase in breast cancer and higher doses of Provera.

Some experts in the medical community have criticized the methodology or size of these studies and argue that they do not support the conclusion of an increased risk.

In other studies, researchers conclude that the progestin actually reduces the risk. Megace, another progestin, has been used for years by oncologists to treat women with metastatic breast cancer. It has been found to extend the survival rate.

The Brain Connection

Turning to the brain, we know that estrogen is important for optimum brain function. I have seen its remarkable effects among my patients. Within an hour or two, a woman with low estrogen is transformed. She goes from having a foggy, unclear mind to enjoying crisp, clear thinking. I know of nothing that works as well as estrogen for this type of transformation.

Your own progesterone also serves the brain. It calms, relaxes, and protects your nervous system. It helps you sleep. It decreases anxiety, depression, and mood swings.

On the other hand, progestins are damaging to nerve cells. They excite and stimulate the nervous system, similar to monosodium glutamate (MSG). They make you nervous and affect your ability to sleep.

For this reason, the use of natural progesterone, not progestins, is advisable.

The Bone Connection

Concerning osteoporosis, progesterone is your best friend. It promotes the buildup of new bone tissue. Estrogen delays the loss of old bone tissue. Together, natural progesterone and estrogen offer major benefits for bone health and can be utilized as powerful weapons against the development of osteoporosis.

I feel that the effect of progesterone on bone health significantly overshadows that of estrogen. I cannot understand why so much emphasis is put on estrogen regarding bone health, while progesterone is ignored.

Depo-Provera, an injectible form of progestin used for birth control, has been found to decrease bone density in young women.

The Diuretic Connection

Progesterone is a beautiful natural diuretic. It prevents the water retention that can be caused by estrogen. If the hormones are in balance, you experience no fluid buildup. With only a few exceptions, water retention is caused by either too much estrogen or too little progesterone.

Progestins, by comparison, cause the body to retain more fluid.

Progestins in the Pipeline

The manufacturers of these products are aware of the problems. And now, with their sights set on the huge female baby boomer market that is perimenopausal and increasingly becoming menopausal, a new generation of progesterone substitutes is being readied to roll onto the market. The new drugs are also called progestins and progestogens, as well as fancier names such as progestomimetics and selective progesterone receptor modulators (SRMs). A few still contain Provera. Most do not. But they are all chemicalized. None of them are the same as the progesterone in your body.

At a January 2000 meeting for physicians in Los Angeles, I listened to a consultant to major pharmaceutical companies describe these up-and-coming products. As I listened I compared the benefits that were being recited to the benefits that my patients get from natural progesterone. And as I listened I also compared the side effects of these patented drugs to the absence of side effects from taking the natural progesterone.

I found that the drugs had few of the major protective benefits of natural progesterone but had a lot of side effects and abnormal reactions.

So why use the drugs?

The manufacturers of these patented, chemicalized hormone substitutes will fund repeated studies to highlight the already well-known benefits, such as protection against uterine cancer. And when the studies are completed, this is what they will publicize and this is what you will hear. I can assure you they will not fund studies to examine the effects of these drugs on the coronary arteries of women.

Through his popular books and newsletters, California physician John Lee, M.D., has done a great service to women by bringing public attention to the benefits of natural progesterone and the dangers of progestins. In the February 2000 issue of his newsletter, Dr. Lee wrote that "using Provera for menopausal women should be considered medical malpractice."

While I share his great concern over the problems associated with this drug, I don't think blame should be directed toward other physicians. It is not their fault. When physicians try to warn patients or take them away from "approved" drugs, they can put their jobs into jeopardy.

Physicians basically respond to the information given them. They receive a great deal of information from pharmaceutical companies. And pharmaceutical companies are the primary sources of advertising revenue for most medical journals read by physicians. Unfortunately, doctors have little or no information about natural hormones. Every other day they see conflicting data on patented, chemicalized hormonal substitutes. They become cynical. They just go with the flow.

Today things are changing. Health care insurers are more sensitive to women's needs and are stepping up their coverage of natural hormones. More information is available today than ever before. Women are talking about natural hormones and asking their physicians.

I am not a wheatgrass eater with an ax to grind. I am not antipharmaceutical. I am just a doctor concerned about the problems with chemicalized hormonal substitutes.

I have three requests to make of the decision makers at the Food and Drug Administration (FDA), where the official approval process takes place:

- Don't allow more new progestins on the market until their potential effects on the coronary arteries and brain and breast tissue are fully investigated.

- Wait until the evidence is in.
- Don't grant fast-track approval until you are sure.

These types of drugs are going to be used by women for many years. Let the manufacturers of these hormonal substitutes prove that they do not increase breast cancer, do not constrict the coronary arteries, and do not have a negative effect on the central nervous system. Be the agency that serves as the protector of women. Fund independent research to test these questions. And if these drugs indeed prove harmful, don't allow them on the market. Don't wait another thirty years until the evidence accumulates that these new drugs, like their predecessors, have the potential to harm the innocent women to whom they are prescribed.

Many articles in popular magazines and women's health newsletters express anger at the media for the uncritical regurgitation of medical reports that fail to distinguish between hormones and their chemicalized substitutes. I don't blame the media. Reporters, unfortunately, don't appear to know the difference. And there is also a tendency in the media to dramatize the findings of medical studies in order to attract more attention.

Many physicians themselves don't know the difference between progesterone and progestins. They haven't been trained to think about options. Many don't even know that natural progesterone is available.

The use of natural progesterone therapy goes back to the pioneering work of Katharina Dalton, M.D., a British physician, who first began using this approach in London fifty years ago. Progesterone treatments have been used in North America since the late 1970s, but only recently have they begun to attract attention because of the fear and dissatisfaction with standard hormonal therapy.

In the late 1980s, Joel Hargrove, M.D., and colleagues at Vanderbilt University's Department of Obstetrics and Gynecology, did a first-of-its-kind comparison of natural progesterone and estradiol with the conventional HRT combination of equine-based estrogen plus progestins. The year-long study involved a small group of menopausal women with moderate to severe symptoms and/or vaginal atrophy.

The Vanderbilt researchers found that the natural combination delivered the same relief of symptoms and protection of uterine tissue, but without any of the adverse effects on blood lipids seen with the use of chemicalized hormones.

The researchers called for larger studies. If the results were duplicated, they suggested, the natural combination could "become the agent of choice" for menopause-related changes because of the poor compliance and acceptance of conventional HRT.

Unfortunately, there have been no larger and longer studies with natural hormones. Makers of hormonal substitutes have no interest in such studies because they would then be promoting products they cannot patent.

If the government will not fund such studies, then it should at least protect us from dangerous drugs. This is a shameful and tragic omission of responsibility. This is where the anger should be vented.

Until something is done, please don't be confused any longer by the medical reports. Progesterone is progesterone, but progestins, progestomimetics, and selective progesterone receptor modulators, are drugs.

13

Basics of Natural Progesterone Replacement

WHAT'S IN THIS CHAPTER

- Prescription and nonprescription progesterone
- Is there a best form?
- Signs of excess progesterone replacement
- The paradoxical progesterone response
- Taking capsules
- Taking sublingual drops
- Using vaginal preparations
- Applying gels and creams
- Taking progesterone and estrogen together

Prescription and Nonprescription Progesterone

Natural progesterone is available in different forms—capsules, gels, sublingual drops, suppositories, and topical and vaginal gels/creams. You can purchase these products from compounding pharmacies. Most regular pharmacies can prepare natural progesterone compounds as well.

The progesterone replacement products I recommend require a doctor's prescription and, similar to estrogen, are available through compounding pharmacies.

Prometrium (capsules) and Crinone (vaginal cream) are two natural products made by pharmaceutical companies. They can be purchased with a prescription from regular pharmacies.

As you probably know, you can obtain progesterone as an over-the-counter cream or gel. Such products are also marketed widely through multi-level and Internet enterprises.

I wish I could be very positive about these creams. The problem is that they have very low concentration—1.5 to 3 percent—and I just haven't seen much evidence of effectiveness among my patients.

Don't be confused by "wild yam extract" products marketed as progesterone. Although wild yams contain compounds from which both progesterone and progestins are chemically processed, your body cannot convert them into progesterone when you eat them.

Is There a Best Form?

The recent entry into the natural progesterone arena of two different products made by pharmaceutical companies has kindled a lively discussion about what form of progesterone is the best. Some experts advocate a topical gel/cream. Others say capsules are better.

According to researchers, when you take progesterone by mouth—in capsule form—the body deactivates 95 percent of it. The deactivation occurs in the liver. Remember, when you take a pill of progesterone, or any medication or vitamin, it enters the digestive tract, is broken down, and then transported directly to the liver. There it is metabolized, meaning that it undergoes a process for further use, storage, or excretion. The substance doesn't pass through the entire circulatory system as it would, for instance, if it were taken sublingually, or applied topically or vaginally.

Remember, I am not a scientist. I am a clinician. I look for results. And I am not concerned if 95 percent is deactivated by the liver. What concerns me is what happens with the active 5 percent. If I see systemic benefits, that means the form is effective.

Researchers also say that the 95 percent deactivated progesterone creates a pool of metabolites with the potential to exert a sedativelike effect. I regard this as a beneficial tool that serves two purposes. One, it helps a woman know if she is taking too much progesterone. And two, many women are glad to have a calming and relaxing effect. For perimenopausal or menopausal women, this is a perfect remedy—a natural tranquilizer—to counteract the sudden anxiety or insomnia that often develops as a result of progesterone deficiency.

In my practice I repeatedly see women smiling again, looking relaxed and rested. Prior to taking progesterone, they were anxious and needed pharmaceutical tranquilizers or sleeping pills.

Advocates of the topical gels and creams say the skin is a superb route for progesterone to enter the body. Yet I find progesterone blood levels of patients using a topical product to be one-tenth that of a patient taking capsules. The fact is that some of the topical gel is metabolized, or deactivated, right in the skin tissue.

Vaginal gels are excellent for concentrating progesterone in the uterus and protecting the endometrium from any pathological thickening. With this method, I see a blood level about one-fifth or one-quarter that of a patient taking capsules.

Each of these progesterone delivery methods offers specific advantages that I take into account when making my recommendations to patients. In the following chapters I will advise you what is the best method for each particular situation.

Signs of Excess Progesterone Replacement

Taking too much progesterone has the potential to cause a few very typical and temporary side effects. Learn to recognize these signs of excess. By doing so, you will quickly master the art of reaching your optimum individual dosage. When and if such reactions occur, you simply reduce the amount of progesterone.

When do reactions occur? Usually within a half hour of taking progesterone. In mild cases, reactions tend not to last more than two hours. If the response is more severe, you can feel the effects for up to eight hours.

There are three types of reactions:

1. Mild Reaction
• Drowsiness.
• Slight dizziness.
• A sense of physical instability.

2. Severe Reaction
• A feeling of being drunk or spinning.
• Heaviness of the extremities.

3. Paradoxical Response
A small percentage of women respond paradoxically to an excess of progesterone hormone replacement. These responses, the opposite of what is

normally expected when someone takes progesterone, are somewhat complex in nature and require a bit of explanation.

The paradoxical effect appears basically to be a reaction among women who can tolerate only a bare minimum of extra progesterone. Here is another example of individuality. For these women, an otherwise normal dosage of progesterone replacement is like a significant overdose. However, even the minimum amount they can tolerate is usually enough to achieve the benefits that would require a much higher dosage in other women.

There are three kinds of paradoxical responses:

- **You feel antsy, anxious, can't sleep, and retain water.** A woman who reacts in this way might, for example, wake up in the middle of the night feeling anxious. This response is believed related to some of the progesterone converting to the antistress hormone cortisol, which in turn could create the agitation.

   The paradoxical occurrence of water retention is likely due to some excess progesterone converting to deoxycorticosterone, a hormone that regulates fluid balance.
- **You experience hot flashes or depression.** In this unusual situation, an excess of progesterone can "down-regulate," or overload, estrogen receptor sites at the cellular level. Less estrogen becomes available to the cells. As a result, signs of estrogen deficiency develop, such as hot flashes or depression. If this occurs, reduce the progesterone.
- **Your appetite increases and you start gaining weight.** This happens only occasionally. I have not found the scientific explanation for it.

Paradoxical responders often have a condition not widely recognized in the conventional medical world: systemic candidiasis. By treating this underlying condition I am usually able to resolve the progesterone paradox among patients. I first put them on a special diet for two weeks that eliminates grains, starches, and sugar.

Next, they start using a low-dose 3 percent progesterone cream, applied vaginally and to the breasts. These are the two critical areas you want to protect. I advise them to slowly increase the amount they apply. Slowly, they increase the strength of the cream and begin applying it elsewhere as well—to the neck, face, and brow, the inner aspects of the arms, and the palms of the hands. I have them change locations frequently but continue applying the cream vaginally and to the breast. If they encounter any side effects, they reduce the amount.

Some women cannot tolerate any increase at all. But sometimes even a minimum quantity is all that's needed to give protection to the breasts and the uterus.

Taking Capsules

Natural progesterone capsules are prepared by a so-called micronization process. This means that progesterone compounds produced in the laboratory are finely ground to enhance absorption and uptake in the body. The smaller the particles, the greater their ability to be absorbed. The fine progesterone powder is then blended with an oil base, which protects it from stomach acid. From the intestines, the progesterone becomes absorbed into the body.

For maximum absorption, take capsules during a meal containing some form of healthy fat. Absorption is not as good on an empty stomach or if the meal contains only carbohydrates.

Oral progesterone enables me to readily obtain a blood level reading. This is important from a clinical standpoint because most of the research in the medical literature links benefits to an optimum blood level range. There are two versions of capsules:

1. Progesterone available through compounding pharmacies that can be tailored to your optimum dosage. This is the form I have been using for many years.

I have found that many of my patients can handle capsules up to 100-milligram strength at night and 50-milligram strength during the day without developing signs of excess. Some have no problem even with much higher doses.

I always recommend progesterone capsules be taken twice a day. Research shows that the supply of progesterone in capsules is used up after twelve hours. *I want twenty-four hours of progesterone protection.* I want it working full-time to benefit not just the uterus, but the bones and the breasts as well, and to create an overall calming effect.

2. Prometrium, a proprietary product developed in Europe from yams. The product was approved by the FDA in late 1999 for use in combination with estrogen drugs for the prevention of endometrial hyperplasia (overgrowth of the uterine lining) in menopausal women. It is available through most regular pharmacies and comes in 100 to 200 milligram potencies.

While I laud this venture by a pharmaceutical company to market a product that contains progesterone structurally identical to the naturally occurring hormone in the body, I find that the currently available potencies are excessive for many women, particularly the higher strength. About a third of my patients find that 100 milligrams is too much.

The manufacturer recommends the pills be taken once a day at bedtime. The rationale is to avoid any daytime drowsiness that might be caused by the high dosage of the hormone if taken in the morning or midday.

A once-a-day dosage is a flawed concept for progesterone replacement. You will lose some of progesterone's protection if you don't take a refill after twelve hours. As I just mentioned, I want a woman to have around-the-clock benefits. That's why I often recommend a smaller morning dose and a larger evening dose. This has the dual purpose of achieving full protection while preventing any possible drowsiness during the day.

In my practice, I prescribe progesterone that patients obtain from compounding pharmacies. This nonproprietary natural progesterone has many more potency options than Prometrium.

If your health insurance plan won't cover nonproprietary natural progesterone, and you don't want to pay out of pocket, you are limited at this time to Prometrium.

When you read the label of Prometrium, don't be shocked. The text is full of the kind of warnings you see on the labels of drugs or birth control pills. I was astounded to see, for instance, "known or suspected pregnancy" as one of the contraindications. Progesterone is one of the main medical tools we have to support pregnancy. The company seems to be treating its product as if it were Provera.

I was also amazed to find a warning on the label about thrombophlebitis, cerebrovascular disorders, and pulmonary embolisms. The risk for these conditions are increased substantially by the use of birth control pills that contain chemicalized hormones. Natural progesterone has no such adverse effect.

The label also mentions malignancy of the breasts or genital organs as contraindications, which is ridiculous. Natural progesterone helps protect the body against cancer.

Any woman reading this label can only be more confused, and more frightened.

I agree with the warning on the label about peanut oil. The manufacturer uses this oil to "deliver" the hormone into the body. Indeed, many people have serious allergies to peanuts and peanut oil.

Strength of Capsules

Natural progesterone capsules are available in potencies of 25, 50, 75, or 100 milligrams.

Taking Sublingual Drops

Drops are well absorbed and handy for most situations. They are particularly useful for PMS, where the dosage may need to be frequently changed.

Administer the drops under the tongue, where they are quickly absorbed into the bloodstream. Wiggle your tongue to enhance the process. Try not to swallow the liquid. If the progesterone drops are swallowed, you lose the benefit of bypassing the liver.

Use a maximum of five or six drops at a time. If you take more, you will have a tendency to swallow some of the progesterone. If your requirements are higher, wait a moment until the first drops are absorbed, and then administer the rest.

Please note that the size of the bottles containing progesterone drops is much larger than estrogen bottles. That's because a larger quantity of progesterone is needed in comparison to estrogen. For this reason, some women find the size inconvenient for carrying during their daily activities.

If the taste of the oil-based drops is unpleasant, you can request the compounding pharmacist to add a natural flavoring such as mint or orange.

Strength of Sublingual Drops

The highest effective concentration currently available is 50 milligrams per eight drops. This is what I use in my practice. I would like an even higher concentration and look forward to this being available through compounding pharmacies in the future. You can obtain a more diluted concentration if you desire, however I see no benefit from it. When I recommend a specific number of drops, please remember that I am referring to drops, not dropperfuls.

Applying Creams and Gels

There are three ways to apply creams and gels. One is vaginally. The second is to the body. The third combines both. I will discuss the first two here. Later, where I discuss specific conditions, I frequently recommend applying creams or gels vaginally as well as topically to the body or breast.

1. The Vaginal Method

Thanks to the pioneering work of Katharina Dalton, M.D., a British physician, natural progesterone first became available to female patients as a suppository in the early 1980s. Between 1982 and 1990 this was the form that I used exclusively for my patients.

Suppositories, and the vaginal creams and gels that came along later, are highly effective for concentrating progesterone in the pelvic area. Recent research with Crinone, a proprietary vaginal gel, has demonstrated the efficiency of the vaginal route for delivering progesterone to the uterus. Studies showed that endometrial concentrations of progesterone are markedly increased with this method in comparison to the oral route.

I recommend vaginal preparations to directly target problems in the uterus, such as fibroids, polyps, or an overgrowth of endometrial tissue, or when patients experience a negative reaction to capsules, topical gels, or sublingual drops. The vaginal route seems to have the lowest potential for unwanted reactions.

The progesterone gel is applied to the "G point," an area at the top of the vagina, just below the uterus. Put a proper amount of the gel onto the tip of a finger. Insert the finger into the vagina and move it straight up, about an inch past the symphysis bone. The "G point" is the creased, wrinkled surface of the upper wall of the vagina. Apply the gel at this spot. Rub it in for a moment. The feedback from my patients is that you will get the maximum absorption there, although absorption is good from anywhere in the vagina.

The vaginal gel is superb for delivering progesterone to the uterus. This method, however, is much less effective in distributing the hormone beyond the pelvic area and through the blood to the rest of the body. According to some studies, the gel generates only a fifth of the progesterone blood level as the oral method.

There is no evidence that the higher concentrations in the uterus, and the lower concentrations in the blood, translate to the benefits you would like to have for the rest of the body. Progesterone is a marvelous substance, with multiple benefits for the whole system, and not just the uterus. I like to extend the zone of protection—to the brain, the breasts, and the bones. Thus, for general use, I prefer other forms of progesterone.

Crinone vaginal gel is another example of a pharmaceutical company making an exact replica of natural human progesterone. However, I am not enchanted with the hydrogenated form of oil used in the preparation. Hydrogenated oils are associated with a type of fatty acid that can be potentially harmful to the body. Still, Crinone gets the job done, and I utilize it if a patient's insurance won't cover the purer compounding pharmacy version.

Strength of gels. I like to use a 10 percent concentration of progesterone. Each gram is equal to a quarter of a teaspoon. Crinone is available in concentrations of 4 or 8 percent.

2. Gels and Creams Applied to the Body

We in the medical community owe John Lee, M.D., a great deal of gratitude for his pioneering research into the benefits of natural progesterone and the use of progesterone cream. Dr. Lee is the author of *What Your Doctor May Not Tell You about Menopause* (Warner Books, 1996).

The attention brought to this method has created some controversy. One of the issues relates to the low, fixed level of progesterone advocated by Dr. Lee. He recommends a 3 percent concentration cream, a potency that is available over-the-counter.

As a clinician, I treat patients and use what is safe and what works. From my experience in treating thousands of patients with a variety of progesterone products, I have found that the low-potency cream is usually not strong enough to resolve the problems I will be discussing here. Here again, I usually prescribe a topical product with 10 percent progesterone concentration.

Progesterone, it turns out, is not absorbed through the skin as well as estrogen. Moreover, a portion of the hormone that is absorbed becomes converted into inactive metabolites in the skin. But if the concentration is strong enough, a topical preparation is a good route for progesterone replacement in spite of the lowered absorption.

Over the years, some of my patients have been influenced by nonmedical health care practitioners to switch to lower-potency over-the-counter creams. I find that they usually lose the benefits previously gained from the higher potency gel I prescribed for them.

Ninety percent of my patients have no problem with the higher potency. For anyone who has a reaction, I reduce the concentration. More than half of my patients experience excellent systemic benefits with the 10 percent gel alone. Others need to take an additional form of progesterone, such as sublingual drops or capsules.

Just as with the estrogen gel, the best areas on the body for absorption are the palms of the hands, the neck, the face and the brow, and the inner

Research shows that the application to the breasts of 10 percent progesterone gel has a significant effect in preventing cell proliferation. For this reason I recommend to patients that for extra protection they apply the gel to the breasts in addition to any other method of using natural progesterone.

arms. Absorption is poor if you apply the progesterone to the abdomen.

Some gels may contain alcohol. They should not be used vaginally. A gel with alcohol can burn vaginal tissue. This is not a problem when applied topically on the skin.

Most of the research on progesterone utilizes blood-level readings. It is important for any physician monitoring your progress to keep in mind that topical application of progesterone, regardless of the potency, always generates a low blood-level value.

Many proponents of low-potency progesterone cream recommend a saliva test to monitor the amount of hormone in the body. I don't regard the test as accurate. It does not help me monitor or fine-tune a patient's hormone level.

Strength of topical creams or gels. Each gram is equal to a quarter of a teaspoon. A 10 percent concentration means each gram contains 100 milligrams of progesterone. You can obtain a lesser concentration, but this level has worked the best for my patients.

TAKING PROGESTERONE AND ESTROGEN TOGETHER

If you opt to take both hormones, as I routinely recommend to patients, the best approach is to start with estrogen alone for a week. Follow my guidelines for estrogen replacement in part two.

In about a week's time, you should be able to develop a good sense of estrogen balance awareness. Once you feel comfortable, then you can start adding progesterone, following the guidelines I will be spelling out in the next three chapters.

14

Natural Progesterone
Replacement for Menopause

WHAT'S IN THIS CHAPTER

- The goal of natural progesterone replacement
- Before starting natural progesterone
- Natural progesterone alone for onset and mid-menopause
- Natural progesterone alone for late menopause
- Combining natural progesterone and estrogen for onset and mid-menopause
- Dose adjustment scenarios
- Combining natural progesterone and estrogen for late menopause
- Monitoring your intake
- Monitoring your intake with your physician

The Goal of Natural Progesterone Replacement

In menopause, your body barely makes any progesterone. However, it is still producing some estrogen. Therefore, a situation of estrogen dominance exists. A progesterone replacement can obviously serve as a first-line weapon against the proliferative effect of unopposed estrogen on the lining of the uterus, but its benefits extend well beyond that. It can do the following for you at this stage of life:

- Reduce much discomfort due to typical menopause-related changes.
- Balance out any possible side effects while you enjoy the benefits of estrogen replacement.

- Eliminate the problems associated with the patented, chemicalized progestin drugs used in conventional replacement therapy.
- Rebuild bone.
- Aid the body's defense system against cancer.
- Decrease water retention.
- Promote relaxation and better sleep.
- Help maintain your proper weight.

In short, progesterone protects you from the side effects of estrogen and maximizes antiaging benefits.

I frequently see new patients who have been taking the typical prescriptive combination of Premarin and Provera. They often complain of being overweight and unable to shed pounds. Their breasts might be twice as large as normal, with much of the enlargement due to water retention. They are anxious. They have difficulty falling asleep. They need Xanax, Valium, Ambien, Halcion, or Tylenol PM for relief.

Just by replacing Provera with natural progesterone, they undergo an almost magical transformation. Their body conformation returns. Their swelling subsides. Their breasts become normal. They are less anxious. They sleep better. And they no longer need their tranquilizers and sleeping aids.

I consistently see these amazing changes. Patients are so relieved that they think I have performed a miracle. I can assure you I am no miracle worker.

All I am doing is introducing them to a hormonal replacement identical to what nature created in their own bodies. The real miracle is the incredible intelligence of the body. I recognize that miracle within and simply try to provide the "right stuff" that reunites a woman with her own inner intelligence.

Again, let me remind you that progesterone and estrogen are complementary. They balance each other. They both need to be there together to form an optimum hormonal partnership, and in this chapter I will teach you how to do it. It's easier than you think. I will, of course, also provide guidelines for those of you who only want to take progesterone alone.

If you have any question about which stage of menopause you fit into, refer back to chapter 8.

Before Starting Natural Progesterone

As is the case with estrogen, there are some preliminary steps I would recommend you do with your physician before starting.

1. Get a pelvic ultrasound to measure your uterine lining. First and foremost, you want to know the status of your endometrial lining. If an excessive thickening has developed, consult with your gynecologist for an evaluation.

The ultrasound also serves to monitor your progress. It will enable your doctor to see firsthand that the natural progesterone offers the same protection to the endometrium as Provera, only without harmful side effects.

2. Have a physical and gynecological checkup, breast exam, and pap smear. If you are over thirty-five, have a mammogram.

Unlike estrogen, you do not need to do a blood test for progesterone before you start replacement. That's because the body has only a minute amount of progesterone at this stage of life.

3. If you plan to take both estrogen and progesterone, start with estrogen first. Refer to my recommendations on estrogen replacement in chapter 8. After developing a good feel for estrogen balance, which shouldn't take more than a few days or a week, begin to add progesterone.

Natural Progesterone Alone for Onset and Mid-Menopause

As I said before, I generally recommend both progesterone and estrogen together. One major reason for this is that estrogen is necessary for the body's utilization of progesterone. Estrogen, and particular estradiol (E2), is intimately involved in the maintenance of cellular progesterone receptor sites.

Hormones are like keys. Receptor sites on the outside and inside of cells are like the locks on doors. Inside the doors are the inner structures of the cells, including the nucleus where the DNA and genetic intelligence respond to messages delivered by hormones.

Estrogen governs the progesterone receptor sites to the cells. So without adequate estrogen on hand, the progesterone key will have fewer locks to open. Less of the progesterone "message" will reach the cells that need it.

Thus, taking progesterone alone in menopause might not be a totally effective strategy.

I have found some patients reluctant to take estrogen. They tend to fit into four categories:

1. Those with a family or personal history of breast cancer.
2. Those interested in progesterone because they have heard it can reduce insomnia.

3. Those interested in progesterone to prevent osteoporosis and also for its other systemic benefits.
4. And women who don't want to take any hormones at all, or just want progesterone.

Refer to the category below that applies to you.

Guidelines for Starting Progesterone for Onset or Mid-Menopause

1. For individuals with a history of breast cancer. Try to attain an optimum level of systemic progesterone using capsules, sublingual drops, or a cream. That means as high a dose as possible without developing any of the signs of excess I described earlier.

Capsules: 50 to 100 milligrams with dinner or before sleep, and 50 milligrams with breakfast or lunch.

Sublingual drops: Eight to sixteen drops before sleep, and four to eight drops at breakfast or lunch. Eight drops is equal to 50 milligrams.

Creams/gels: Apply 1 gram of the 10 percent cream twice a day to the neck, face and brow, or inner side of the arms, or the palms.

In addition, I recommend applying progesterone directly to the breasts once a day. Recent studies have shown that such application of a 10 percent progesterone cream counteracts the proliferation of breast tissue caused by estrogen. As a result, one European study of forty menopausal women concluded, progesterone "may protect against hyperplasia." Hyperplasia is a medical term for tissue overgrowth.

Among this group I give lesser importance to the use of vaginal cream. While this is a powerful method for delivering progesterone to the uterus and the pelvic cavity, it appears less effective for a wider distribution of the hormone throughout the body.

2. For better sleep and anxiety reduction. Insomnia during menopause primarily relates to estrogen deficiency. Yet, if you don't want to take an estrogen replacement, you often can use a high dosage of progesterone to give you a restful night's sleep. Based on my experience with patients, I estimate that three-quarters of women could probably resolve a hormonal-related sleeping problem with this simple approach.

Research in Germany has shown that progesterone has neuropsychopharmacological properties. This scientific term means that it has a potent effect on brain chemistry. Specifically, it enhances the activity of GABA, a major neurochemical that calms the nervous system. Researchers have found that progesterone produces a sleep brain wave pattern similar to that from tranquilizers.

Your strategy is to optimize the dosage and capitalize on this function of progesterone. Take the maximum amount that is comfortable for you before sleep. Take a lesser amount in the morning or at midday. Capsules or drops work the best here.

Capsules or sublingual drops: Start with two 50-milligram strength capsules (for a total of 100 milligrams) taken in bed a half hour before bedtime.

If you prefer drops, start with eight. But don't take more than six drops at a time. Wait a moment, and then add the remaining drops.

If the starting dosage doesn't work, increase the amount you take by an additional 50-milligram capsule, or four drops, on subsequent evenings. Stop increasing once you experience a full night of restful sleep or if you develop side effects from excess progesterone. Such side effects include increased water retention, a depressed feeling, or waking up groggy or edgy.

Earlier in the day, at breakfast or lunch, take a 50-milligram capsule, or four to six sublingual drops. Be alert to the fact that there may be some residual progesterone in the body in the morning and you might experience some drowsiness if you take the hormone with breakfast. Remember that the effectiveness of progesterone capsules or drops lasts for up to twelve hours in your system. With a bit of experimentation, you will quickly be able to determine your optimum dose and schedule. Taking progesterone with lunch may work better for you than breakfast.

Some women cannot tolerate a dose at either breakfast or lunch. If you are such a person, taking progesterone before bedtime will probably be enough to do the job for you.

Some women are able to tolerate a very high dosage of progesterone—up to about 300 milligrams at a time. Few can tolerate more. My wife is one of those few. She can handle up to 400 or 500 milligrams without a problem.

If you need some calming and reduction of anxiety in your life, progesterone's natural sedative effect can be of great benefit. The strategy of maximum progesterone at night and a lesser dose earlier in the day is helpful for most women.

When this strategy doesn't work and your anxiety level is still higher than you would like it to be, try taking smaller and more frequent doses throughout the day. You may get relief with 25- or 50-milligram capsules four times a day, such as at breakfast, lunch, midafternoon, and dinner. Don't be afraid to experiment. Just watch for signs of excess, and if they develop, reduce your dosage.

Always keep in mind the individuality factor.

3. For preventing osteoporosis. Progesterone is an unheralded protector of female bones. The hormone stimulates new bone cell growth and at the same time promotes old bone cell removal.

By comparison, estrogen slows down both the growth of new bone tissue formation and the removal of old bone.

Recognition of the beneficial role of progesterone has been lost in the calcium mania that permeates our society. *Some researchers have even suggested that menopausal osteoporosis may be in part a progesterone deficiency disease.* For sure, we need more research here and also to bring the bone-building promise of progesterone to women's attention.

Capsules or sublingual drops. 100 to 150 milligrams in capsule form, or eight to twelve drops, at bedtime. Take a 50-milligram capsule, or six drops, with breakfast or lunch.

Creams/gels. Applying 10 percent progesterone gel or cream to the designated areas on the body is optional.

4. For women who don't want to take any hormones, or who just want progesterone. I sincerely believe that every woman in menopause should take at least progesterone. Progesterone provides balance against unopposed estrogen, and every woman in menopause has some degree of unopposed estrogen, even if it is minor. Remember, the body is still making some estrogen.

Unopposed estrogen can increase the risk of breast and uterine cancer. Medical studies show this clearly. You can eliminate or reduce the risk with progesterone.

However, if you take progesterone alone, be aware that estrogen maintains the cellular receptor sites for progesterone. Progesterone alone could block some of this estrogen function. That could actually inhibit some of the ability of progesterone to perform its job inside the cells.

Creams/gels. Apply 10 percent progesterone cream to the breasts twice a day. Why 10 percent and not the low-dose creams available over-the-counter? All the medical studies showing benefit to breast tissue were conducted using this concentration. There is no evidence of benefits to the breast with lower potencies.

Vaginal cream. Crinone cream (4 or 8 percent potencies) once a day has been shown to provide endometrial protection.

You can also use 1 gram of 10 percent progesterone cream once or twice a day for similar protection.

Natural Progesterone Alone for Late Menopause

For this stage of menopause, I recommend a lower potency gel or cream—3 percent concentration. Apply it topically twice a day. Follow the guidelines for gels in the previous chapter. Gradually increase the strength of the gel to 10 percent.

Progesterone will protect you from possible harmful effects caused by the remaining unopposed estrogen in your body. In addition, it will calm and relax you, and contribute to better sleep.

Combining Natural Progesterone and Estrogen for Onset and Mid-Menopause

In my opinion, everyone should use this combined approach. The benefits are multiplied. And you will be surprised how simple it is to balance the two hormones.

The easiest way to start, and particularly if you experience many estrogen fluctuations at the onset of menopause, is to keep your estrogen and progesterone replacements separate.

Start with estrogen first. Adjust your dosage by following the guidelines I spelled out earlier. Once you are comfortable and have a good handle on adjusting your estrogen, start adding progesterone. And once the estrogen fluctuations disappear, you may like to combine the estrogen and progesterone in a single capsule, gel, or liquid product.

Guidelines for Starting and for Individuals Switching from Conventional Hormonal Replacement Therapy

For progesterone, use the following amounts:

Capsules. 50 to 100 milligrams with dinner or before sleep, and 50 to 100 milligrams with breakfast or lunch.

Sublingual drops. Eight to twelve drops before sleep, and four to six drops at breakfast or lunch.

To determine your starting dose of estrogen, refer back to chapter 8.

If, after starting to combine the two hormones, you experience water retention, bloating, or breast tenderness, the cause could be not enough progesterone or too much estrogen. How do you figure what the problem is?

The first thing to do is try increasing the progesterone in order to reach an optimum level.

What if you increase the progesterone and develop signs of excess? That means you have reached your optimum dose for progesterone. You can't bump it up anymore. Now you have to consider the cause may be too much estrogen.

The next step would be to decrease the estrogen. That often solves the problem.

What if reducing estrogen doesn't resolve the problem and it creates instead signs of estrogen deficiency such as night sweats and hot flashes?

Now what?

You can't take more progesterone and you can't decrease the estrogen.

Don't be concerned. What's happened here is simple. There are two estrogen players in the game. One is the estrogen replacement and the other is the estrogen still being produced in your body.

At this point in menopause, there are still some fluctuations of estrogen. You have probably caught a temporary upward fluctuation that caused the water retention, bloating, or breast tenderness. Remember that it takes a few days for signs of excess estrogen to be felt. It is unlikely that the symptoms will last very long. So simply ride them out and continue with the regular doses of your hormones.

Creams/gels: Many women prefer this form. To save money or for convenience, they often like to combine estrogen and progesterone in one cream. I don't recommend an all-in-one combination at the start. A combined hormone product makes it very difficult, if not impossible, to adjust individual hormones and deal with estrogen fluctuations. So I advise two separate products that can be adjusted as needed. When fluctuations stop, or you find that you are using the same amount consistently, that's the time to think about combining.

Start with 10 percent progesterone gel. Apply 1 gram (one-quarter teaspoon) twice daily, in the morning and evening. For perhaps 90 percent of women, this dosage creates a healthy and desirable thinning of the uterus lining.

In the remaining cases, the topical gel doesn't give enough protection to the uterus. You can, of course, also apply it vaginally. Just be sure it contains no alcohol. To confirm that you are not among the small percentage of women who does not respond, I recommend monitoring with pelvic ultrasound once a year or whenever there is an episode of vaginal bleeding.

For women who don't tolerate the 10 percent gel/cream, request the compounding pharmacist to make you a weaker prescription. But be sure to apply the progesterone to the breasts and vagina as well. Lowering the potency reduces the possibility of side effects while giving protection to the most critical areas.

Dose Adjustment Scenarios
JOYCE'S STORY

Joyce, forty-nine, was menopausal for six months. She had used the combination of Premarin-Provera for three months. Then she stopped because of unwanted weight gain and increase in breast size. On her first visit to my office, she complained of nervousness and difficulty falling asleep.

After an evaluation, I recommended Tri-Est gel and progesterone capsules. Joyce balanced herself fairly quickly. About five months later she called and asked what to do about severe breast tenderness that had developed.

I told her initially to increase her progesterone before sleep from 100 to 150 milligrams, and see if she could also raise her midday dose from 50 to 100 milligrams. She found she could add the 50 milligrams at night, but not during the day without feeling some slight drowsiness in the afternoon. However, the additional progesterone in the evening didn't reduce her breast tenderness.

I now suggested she decrease her estrogen intake by 25 percent, from 1 gram to $3/4$ gram twice a day. She immediately experienced hot flashes, a sign of estrogen deficiency.

It now became apparent that Joyce was having one of those temporary surges in estrogen that was causing the breast tenderness. I assured her that the discomfort would only last for a few days. I advised her to ride it out and resume her regular hormone replacement dosages. She followed my instructions. In a few days she called to report that all was back to normal.

Joyce's story is interesting because it dramatizes a common situation where the body produces a short-term burst of estrogen in early menopause. It takes about four or five days before you feel the effects of excess.

Initially, I thought the problem might be related to insufficient progesterone. That's why I had her raise the dosage of progesterone. That didn't help her. So the next step was to lower the level of estrogen. Maybe she was taking too much. That didn't work either. She quickly developed hot flashes. Then it was obvious she was going through a temporary surge in estrogen production, an upward fluctuation. Usually, these estrogen spikes last only a few days and then the level drops again. And indeed, this was Joyce's experience.

GINA'S STORY

Gina, fifty-two, one year in menopause, was using 100 milligrams of progesterone at night, 50 in the morning, as well as taking three Tri-Est sublingual drops twice a day.

She called, complaining of breast tenderness and water retention. She was having trouble getting into her shoes, taking her rings on and off, and felt bloated.

"I try to decrease the estrogen from three to two drops, but when I do I get hot flashes," she said. "I can't seem to find a happy medium. Either I have hot flashes or tender breasts."

"Try adding 50 milligrams of progesterone at night and also at lunch," I suggested.

Initially she felt better. But within a week she complained of hot flashes again, more water retention, and a slight depression. She was more confused.

I interpreted her reaction as a result of too much progesterone. She had, in fact, developed a paradoxical reaction to progesterone, an unusual response that I described in chapter 13. The excess progesterone was blocking her estrogen receptors. This effect decreased the effectiveness of her estrogen replacement and is why she developed hot flashes and depression. In addition, the excess progesterone had interfered with the function of a related hormone that regulates body fluids. This caused the water retention.

Her predicament was this: if she reduced her estrogen, she developed hot flashes and signs of estrogen deficiency. If she took more progesterone, she developed the paradoxical response.

The only solution for her was to maintain her regular level of estrogen and progesterone, and apply a 10 percent progesterone cream to the breasts. This approach provided her breasts with extra protection from the cream while reducing the water retention. Critically for her, it did not raise the overall progesterone level in her body enough to cause problems. Keep in mind that the absorption of progesterone through the skin is much less than through the oral method.

I probably would have been able to achieve the same results by adding 25 milligrams of progesterone orally.

SHARON'S STORY

Sharon, fifty-three, was menopausal. She made an appointment with me in order to switch from conventional HRT to natural hormones. I put her on a program of estrogen gel and progesterone sublingual drops.

A month later she returned to tell me how good she felt on the natural hormones.

"My breasts are less tender, my mind is clearer, I feel less edgy, and I am actually losing weight," she said.

But she wanted me to help her fine-tune her hormones.

"Anytime I try to increase the amount of gel in order to get more relief, I do great for a few days," she explained. "But then I feel the tenderness return to my breasts. So I have to return to using less gel again. If I try to take more progesterone, I become sleepy in the middle of the day. It starts about a half hour after I take the progesterone and can last for a couple of hours."

I then explained that what she was experiencing was a physiological effect from a decrease in her sex hormone–binding globulin.

"With Premarin," I said, "your sex hormone–binding globulin level was very high. Remember that when you take estrogen orally, it raises your level of this protein that regulates the amount of hormones available in your body. The additional sex hormone–binding globulin binds up some of the estrogen you are taking, along with other hormones. So you wind up having to take more estrogen in order to get the desired benefits. Now, with the use of the gel, the level of your sex hormone–binding globulin decreases. It will take six to eight weeks. And as long as it stays at the lower level, you will find you need less estrogen replacement."

I told her that her body was very responsive and that in a few weeks she would come to a point where the need to adjust would be only minimal.

Combining Natural Progesterone and Estrogen for Late Menopause

Guidelines for Starting

To determine your starting dose of estrogen, refer back to chapter 8.

Here is how to add progesterone:

Creams/gels: Start with 1 gram (one-quarter teaspoon) at 3 percent strength, applied twice daily. Over time you can increase the potency. Go up to 6 percent, and then 10 percent, if desired.

Capsules: Start with 25 milligrams, at breakfast or lunch, and again before bedtime.

After you become accustomed to the progesterone, increase your morning or lunch dose to a maximum of 50 milligrams and to 100 milligrams in the evening, if desired. If you raise the evening dose, do it very slowly, first going to 50, then 75, and then 100 milligrams.

In the beginning, or whenever you increase the potency of your evening dosage, wait until you are in bed to take the capsule. As I have mentioned, progesterone has the potential to cause some drowsiness or even dizziness. For this reason it is prudent to take it at bedtime and not when you are up and active. You want to avoid any risk of falling, even if it is a remote possibility.

Guidelines for Switching from Conventional Hormonal Replacement Therapy

At this stage, women do not tolerate sublingual drops or the vaginal type of creams.

Creams/gels: Start with ½ gram (one-eighth of a teaspoon) of 10 percent progesterone twice daily for a few days. Apply to body as I have suggested. If tolerated, increase to a quarter teaspoon twice a day.

Capsules: Starting and maintenance doses are 50 milligrams at lunch and 100 milligrams at bedtime.

Monitoring Your Intake

It's very simple. You are taking an adequate amount of progesterone when you achieve any of the following results:

- Decreased water retention
- Reduced breast tenderness
- You're feeling more relaxed
- You're sleeping better.

Remember, if you experience breast tenderness or enlargement, or water retention, and you reduce your estrogen level and encounter signs of estrogen deficiency, that means that you can generally use more progesterone. But if you can't take more progesterone by increasing the potency of the capsules or adding more sublingual drops, then apply the progesterone gel to the breasts. If that gives you only partial relief, then also apply the gel vaginally.

Monitoring Your Intake with Your Physician

Request a pelvic ultrasound once a year to monitor the status of the endometrial lining. You want to see a thin lining, no more than five millimeters thick. If it is thicker, you should have a gynecological evaluation.

If the progesterone provides adequate protection against tissue proliferation in the uterus, it should also protect the breasts.

If you use a vaginal progesterone cream, keep in mind that this type of product concentrates the hormone in the uterus and probably won't give much effective protection elsewhere in the body, including the breasts.

To monitor your hormonal level, your blood should be drawn six to eight hours after taking or applying the progesterone.

You want to see a hormonal value ranging from 5 to 25 ng/ml, if you use capsules or drops. For topical gels, the values are much lower because absorption is not as good. Usually the level is 1 or 2 ng/ml, and rarely more than 3.

For women who use vaginal creams only, a peak level occurs two hours after application. A good level is in the 4 or 5ng/ml range.

Interpretations of estrogen blood levels have been described earlier. It is important to maintain as constant a level of estrogen as possible.

15

Natural Progesterone Replacement for Perimenopause

WHAT'S IN THIS CHAPTER

- The goal of natural progesterone replacement
- Before starting natural progesterone
- How to take natural progesterone for perimenopause
- If you are switching from Provera or the birth control pill
- Monitoring your intake
- Monitoring your intake with your physician
- What about adding estrogen?

The Goal of Natural Progesterone Replacement

In my opinion, every woman in perimenopause should take progesterone. The hormonal irregularities at this stage of life can last anywhere from three months to ten years. Progesterone can play a powerful role in smoothing out the hormonal bumps and jolts.

Starting in the midthirties, and sometimes earlier, progesterone production starts to wane. Compared to earlier peak years, the level in your body varies from low to extremely low by the time you reach perimenopause.

Dwindling progesterone is the central cause for the upsetting irregularity of the bleeding pattern. And with less and less progesterone on hand to balance estrogen, the hormonal drama that now unfolds in your body becomes an increasingly solo performance of soaring and plunging estrogen. One moment you may have symptoms of estrogen excess, the next moment of estrogen deficiency. In either case, estrogen is dominant. You lack balance.

The aim of hormonal replacement now is to regain balance by replenishing progesterone. Restored balance helps your body fight cancer, achieve optimum health, and prevent a range of bleeding abnormalities that are considered indications for surgery.

You could argue that it is not natural for a woman to have progesterone replaced at this time. Why go against the body's own biological script?

It's a good question. Let me answer by citing four ways to approach the issue of progesterone replacement at perimenopause.

1. The Do-Nothing Approach

Let nature do its job, many women say. But nature never really counted on you living so long. Now, at perimenopause or beyond, your body has only estrogen and little progesterone for balance. As a consequence, you may experience abnormal bleeding and fibroids, and an increased risk of uterine cancer and unnecessary surgery. All these can be avoided, or reduced in frequency, with natural progesterone replacement.

2. Birth Control Pills

Increasingly, women are prescribed the pill in order to create monthly regularity and prevent abnormal bleeding.

I disagree with this approach. In the first place, you are likely to develop side effects from the chemicalized progestin in the pill. Secondly, the estrogen in the pill is exclusively an aggressive form of chemicalized estrogen.

Thirdly, the additional estrogen could stimulate the liver to produce more sex hormone–binding globulin. This results in a reduction of your already dwindling antiaging hormones.

3. Provera

Take Provera ten days or two weeks out of the month. I have already described my serious reservations about this drug.

4. Give Back to the Body What It Needs and Thrives On

You and your body will thrive with real progesterone.

Before Starting Natural Progesterone

Prior to starting progesterone replacement, obtain a pelvic ultrasound to rule out the presence of endometrial tissue overgrowth. Perimenopause means your body has been in estrogen dominance for months or even years.

In my clinical experience, endometrial overgrowth can be reversed in the great majority of cases with progesterone, even if a significant buildup of tissue has developed and reached a precancerous state.

However, if ultrasound determines such an overgrowth, be sure to follow your doctor's advice for treatment.

How to Take Natural Progesterone for Perimenopause

Use any systemic form of progesterone (capsules, sublingual drops, or topical creams/gels) continually twice a day for two weeks of the month. You can organize this according to your cycle, from day fifteen to day twenty-eight, or if your cycle is too irregular, then choose any day of the month and take that as your starting point. For example, you might use progesterone from the first of the month to the fifteenth, or from the fifteenth to the thirtieth.

Challenge your body. I suggest using as much progesterone as you can tolerate without any sign of excess. Follow the guidelines in onset menopause. The only difference is that for perimenopause you will take progesterone for only two weeks out of the month.

Although you will be reestablishing cyclicity, keep in mind that irregularities may occur because of the unpredictable fluctuations of your estrogen. The amount of bleeding is dictated by your estrogen activity. One month you may have a heavy flow, the next month no flow, and the next month a minimum flow.

If any buildup in endometrial tissue is diagnosed through pelvic ultrasound after starting your replacement program, apply a vaginal progesterone cream in addition to the systemic form of progesterone. Use a 10 percent cream once or twice daily. This will effectively deliver the hormone to the uterus and reduce the overgrowth. Refer to my guidelines in chapter 13 for applying vaginal creams.

If You Are Switching from Provera or the Birth Control Pill

Follow my recommendations in the previous chapter for onset menopause women who are starting progesterone. Again, the only difference here is that you take progesterone for only two weeks out of the month.

The pill suppresses your own estrogen and progesterone production.

When you stop the pill, it takes a few months or more before the body is able to resume making the hormones normal again.

Once you have used progesterone for a few cycles, have your estradiol and FSH levels checked. If the results show you to be deficient in estrogen, then refer back to chapter 8.

Monitoring Your Intake

Here is what you can expect to see from replacement with natural progesterone:

- A more regular period
- More calmness
- Improved sleep
- Reduced water retention.

Women with high estrogen production can expect long, full periods. The high level of estrogen promotes endometrial tissue growth, so higher-than-usual sloughing will occur.

In these situation, I try to counterbalance the estrogen buildup by increasing the dosage of progesterone as much as possible without causing any discomfort.

Women with a lower than average amount of estrogen will experience a smaller amount of bleeding when progesterone is used. Less estrogen generates less endometrial tissue growth. This means you will see less sloughing. During some periods there may be no bleeding at all.

Women with very low estrogen, and who have signs of estrogen deficiency, will not have another period after starting progesterone.

Different reactions to the progesterone at perimenopause call for different strategies. I classify them as "the four ifs." (See page 141.)

In my practice, many perimenopausal patients feel so good after they start progesterone that they want to take the hormone continually and not just for two weeks of the month.

More than half of those who do so receive all the feel-good and protective influences of progesterone throughout the whole month. Among others, however, continual administration leads to a new type of irregularity: frequent light bleeding.

You can avoid this by taking the progesterone for the first two weeks of the month at night only and the rest of the month twice a day. Or, take the pro-

THE FOUR IFS

If No. 1

If you spot occasionally while taking progesterone, don't pay attention, and simply continue taking it.

If No. 2

If you repeatedly spot or get your period before the end of the two weeks on progesterone, that's a clue to take more of the hormone. Raise your level as high as you can tolerate without any side effects. If these symptoms are hormonally based, adding progesterone will create the balance to eliminate them. If you maximize your dosage to the highest level you can tolerate and still do not experience regularity, you should consult with your physician. You may have a condition developing in the uterus, such as polyps, fibroids, or adenomyosis.

If No. 3

If, while taking the progesterone, you experience a heavy flow of blood, stop the progesterone. Consider this to be the first day of a new cycle. Resume the hormone two weeks later.

If No. 4

If your period doesn't come within a week after you stopped taking the progesterone, consider the last day you took progesterone as day one of a new cycle. Resume the progesterone two weeks from that date.

gesterone for twenty to twenty-two days of the month, and then skip a week. If you can't regulate the bleeding, and it is annoying you, then go back to the sequential pattern of two weeks on and two weeks off.

Monitoring Your Intake with Your Physician

If you started with an abnormally thick endometrium, a pelvic ultrasound should confirm a return to normal within a few cycles after starting progesterone.

To measure the progesterone level in the blood, have a blood sample drawn six to eight hours after taking the hormone. Refer to the criteria on page 136 (in the menopause chapter) on interpreting the results.

You may not be able to correct irregular and unpredictable bleeding in the presence of adenomyosis, a condition involving abnormal endometrial growth into the deeper level of uterine muscle tissue. Even your best efforts with progesterone and the help of your physician may fail.

What about Adding Estrogen?

After starting on progesterone for two weeks of the month, you will probably wonder what is going on with your estrogen.

Assess how you feel. Your subjective experience from taking progesterone gives you a yardstick for the status of your estrogen level.

1. You have a proper amount of estrogen if you bleed normally.
2. You have a lower amount of estrogen than you had in the past if you have reduced bleeding, or don't bleed at all. Less endometrial tissue is growing and there is thus less tissue to slough. From a physiological perspective, as long as you bleed less than before, or not at all, your body isn't producing the same amount of estrogen as in the past. But always take individuality into account. Some patients tell me that even if they don't bleed or just bleed slightly, they have no evidence of estrogen deficiency. In this situation, they usually have no need, or desire, to take estrogen. If there are any signs of deficiency, regardless of how much they bleed, I suggest taking estrogen. In perimenopause, women shouldn't have to get to the point where they become fatigued, develop foggy minds, have difficulty falling asleep, or lose their zest for life before replacing estrogen.
3. Monitor yourself more closely if you take progesterone, are not bleeding, and start to notice the obvious signs of estrogen deficiency. You could be going through temporary fluctuations of low estrogen lasting weeks or months. Or you may be entering into menopause. In either case, you may want to consider estrogen replacement. For more information, refer back to chapter 9 on perimenopause and estrogen.
4. Some women experience unpredictable cycles of heavy, slight, or no bleeding. This tells you that your estrogen is constantly fluctuating.

16

Natural Progesterone Replacement for Younger Women

Who Should Take Natural Progesterone?

Any woman who does not follow the natural design of multiple cycles of pregnancy and breast-feeding has some degree of estrogen dominance. For this reason, I would prefer to see women taking progesterone for balance and added protection, even when they are younger. Such a vision, of course, is idealistic. But from a practical standpoint, there are certain groups of younger women who can obtain great benefit and relief with natural progesterone. These women are the subject of this chapter.

143

Women Who Have no Periods (Amenorrhea)

There are two possible conditions involved:

1. Primary amenorrhea, where a woman has never had a period.
2. Secondary amenorrhea, where a woman has had periods but stops ovulating for at least six months.

Let's consider each separately and how progesterone can help.

Primary Amenorrhea

There is no ovulation. The body does not produce an adequate amount of estrogen, and the level of progesterone is minimal.

These deficiencies can be objectively confirmed through blood tests. The tests will show low levels of estrogen, progesterone, FSH, and sex hormone–binding globulin.

Progesterone and estrogen replacements are both needed.

The guiding principle to progesterone replacement is whether or not you want a period. Some women feel something is missing from their lives unless they menstruate. Some don't care. From a purely medical standpoint, there is no benefit to having a period.

Secondary Amenorrhea

Secondary amenorrhea occurs frequently during the first year of menstruation, prior to perimenopause, among women with thyroid disorder, and among those who have stopped taking the birth control pill. The body barely makes progesterone. There is no ovulation.

Estrogen and SHBG are normal. Obviously, this is a situation of significant estrogen dominance.

Most women with primary or secondary amenorrhea are prescribed birth control pills as the treatment of choice because it *allegedly* restores the normality of the period. Anytime a woman takes the birth control pill she will get regular periods. But the hormonal balance you think has been achieved is really a bogus and harmful imitation of balance. You have actually created a new predicament. First, the pill eliminates the chance that the body will restore balance on its own, and two, it aggravates estrogen dominance. These women need both estrogen and progesterone, or progesterone alone. We should be replacing what they need and not dumping chemicalized hormonal substitutes into their bodies that totally depress their systems.

Natural Progesterone for Primary Amenorrhea

In chapter 10 I discussed how women without periods can remedy their situation with estrogen. Progesterone enters the equation if you want to achieve regular menstruation.

In order to produce bleeding, you take progesterone two weeks out of the month, starting on the fifteenth day of the cycle. Then you stop. If your body has enough estrogen, the period should follow.

I try to steer young women away from this practice because it perpetuates a "part-time" estrogen dominance. The remainder of the month you will have no progesterone protection against estrogen. For this reason, I recommend to patients that they take progesterone throughout the month.

You may want to consider this option for the continual protection and balance that progesterone offers. I discussed the pros and cons of this approach in the last chapter. Refer to the section on monitoring your intake.

Capsules: 50 to 150 milligrams at bedtime or dinner, and 50 milligrams with lunch or breakfast. Capsules work the best here. Follow the guidelines in chapter 14 for starting with progesterone in onset menopause.

Primary Amenorrhea: Monitoring Your Intake

If you have enough estrogen, you will always experience menstruation after supplementing with progesterone for two weeks.

If you have a very heavy flow, you may be using too much estrogen.

If you have a very slight period, such as a few spots, you may not be using enough estrogen. But if you feel well, don't increase the estrogen.

If you have no period, along with signs of estrogen deficiency, you definitely need more estrogen.

In principle, if there is enough estrogen on board, you will have a period after two weeks of taking progesterone.

Probably 90 percent of those who take estrogen and progesterone daily will not experience bleeding. The rest will bleed intermittently and not in a predictable fashion. In the long run, most individuals who are balanced will stop bleeding.

Primary Amenorrhea: Monitoring Your Intake with Your Physician

Have a blood test two or three months after you start the program. You'll be checking your levels of estradiol, progesterone, and sex hormone–binding globulin. The blood should be taken during the time of the month you use both estrogen and progesterone. The time for the draw is six to eight hours after taking the hormones.

You want to see estradiol between 50 and 250 pg/ml, progesterone over 5 ng/ml, and SHBG under 90 nmol/l.

If your estradiol level is very low, a sign that you don't have enough estrogen, you won't get a period. The fact that you get your period means that both hormones are doing what they are supposed to do. So don't get totally fixated on the numbers in the test. Get in tune with what is going on in your body.

If estradiol and SHBG are higher than the values I just mentioned, you should reduce the amount of estrogen, or switch from estrogen capsules or drops to a gel.

If your progesterone level is low (below 5) after four or five months of replacement, you should have a pelvic ultrasound test. The time to have the ultrasound is following the end of your period (if you have a period) or any time of the month (if you don't have a period). You are right on track with the program if the lining of the uterus is normal.

Natural Progesterone for Secondary Amenorrhea

Capsules or sublingual drops: Follow my guidelines for progesterone at perimenopause in the previous chapter. Take twice daily two weeks out of the month. This follows the normal pattern of the body's production. I have found that gels or creams, even at 10 percent strength, are not always effective enough to create regular cyclicity.

Secondary Amenorrhea: Monitoring Your Intake. Your program is effective if you achieve a regular cycle and have no signs of PMS.

Secondary Amenorrhea: Monitoring Your Intake with Your Physician

After two or three months on the program, check the progesterone level between day nineteen to twenty-one. The best time of the day for the test is about three hours after taking progesterone in the morning. Remember what I said about anything over 15 ng/ml being considered the optimum range. That's where you want to see your level as long as you have no signs of excessive progesterone.

Let's say you are successful in achieving your goal of regularity and control of bleeding. You have no side effects of excess progesterone. And now your physician says your level of progesterone is too high. Don't be concerned. Explain that the test has measured a peak level of progesterone, three hours after taking the hormone. If you were to measure it later in the afternoon, the level would be lower by a third or even half.

If you cannot achieve regularity with progesterone within two or three cycles, I recommend you see your gynecologist in order to rule out any possible problems such as polyps, fibroids, or endometrial tissue overgrowth.

Women with Abnormal Bleeding

If a young woman has abnormal bleeding we first want to rule out pregnancy. If she is not pregnant, we want to determine whether or not she is ovulating.

In this section I want to concentrate on women who ovulate yet produce insufficient progesterone after ovulation. This situation results in two different bleeding patterns:

1. A normal flow occurring earlier in the monthly cycle. Instead of every twenty-eight days, the full period usually begins anywhere from day eighteen to twenty-six.
2. Spotting before the period for a few days or even up to a week.

In medical terms, we refer to these situations as corpus luteum insufficiency. The corpus luteum is the section of the ovaries where progesterone is produced and which nourishes the embryo in the first few weeks of pregnancy.

These patterns of abnormal bleeding can occur in women ranging from teenagers to individuals in their forties and early fifties. The patterns are most frequent during the first five years of menstruation and over the age of thirty-five. They are related to the characteristic cyclic fall of progesterone after ovulation. If the fall is sharp and steep, a full period develops earlier than usual. If the fall happens earlier than normal, spotting develops prior to the usual onset of menstruation.

You can pretty much gauge the degree of progesterone deficiency in the following way. The greater your deficiency the quicker the onset of bleeding after ovulation. The earlier that spotting occurs, the earlier the drop of progesterone in your cycle.

You can verify ovulation with an ovulation prediction test, a device available in pharmacies.

Natural Progesterone for Abnormal Bleeding

Your aim is to restore regularity and prevent spotting and early menstruation. The problem results from not enough progesterone.

If you suffer from PMS, refer to my guidelines later in this chapter for PMS.

If you don't have a PMS problem, take progesterone from day fifteen to day twenty-eight of the cycle. If your cycle is abnormally short, take the hormone for two weeks following the day you ovulate. Choose one of the following methods:

Capsules: 100 milligrams at dinner or before sleep, 50 milligrams at breakfast or lunch.

Sublingual drops: Eight to twelve drops before sleep, four to eight drops in the morning or midday.

Topical cream: Apply a 10 percent strength cream, starting with 1/2 gram twice daily for the first week, and then 1 gram twice daily afterward.

Contrary to advertising claims, I have found that low-potency over-the-counter progesterone creams are usually not strong enough to do the job. The few who do respond tend to have a very minimal deficiency. If these creams cannot restore the regularity of the period due to low progesterone, I wonder how much they can provide for other progesterone-related functions in the body.

Often, and particularly among women in their late thirties and forties where the deficiency worsens, even 10 percent progesterone cream may not resolve the problem.

Vaginal cream. Apply 10 percent strength twice daily or Crinone 4 or 8 percent cream once a day.

Monitoring Your Intake

With proper administration of progesterone you should be able to resolve the problem of abnormal bleeding.

If you don't achieve your objective in the first cycle, and you still spot or bleed prematurely, increase the level of progesterone in the next cycle, especially after day twenty-one.

If the amount you need to achieve regularity creates side effects, then decrease the amount of the capsules or drops you are using. Add a 10 percent vaginal progesterone cream to your routine.

In case these strategies don't work, your problem may not be progesterone deficiency. You should see your gynecologist for an evaluation.

Monitoring Your Intake with Your Physician

See comments under secondary amenorrhea on pages 146–47.

Women with PMS

Premenstrual syndrome was first described in medical terms by a New York endocrinologist in 1931. It involves an array of physical and emotional symptoms that develop after ovulation and before the onset of the period. Symptoms vary from woman to woman. Sometimes they start a day or two before the period. Sometimes two weeks before. Sometimes the intensity is mild. At other times, it is significant enough to be debilitating. PMS usually intensifies gradually as you get closer to your period.

Research has linked the stressful physiological and psychological symptoms to a decline in circulating progesterone. In recent years, scientific investigators have found mounting evidence of a strong relationship between progesterone and GABA, a major brain neurotransmitter that produces a calming effect throughout the nervous system. Progesterone enhances GABA. When progesterone is deficient, anxiety and PMS symptoms can result.

In my clinical experience, PMS can be eliminated or significantly improved in about 95 percent of patients with a combined nutritional supplement and progesterone program. I will describe both of these approaches in this section. The remaining small percentage of women who do not entirely respond have an estrogen deficiency that also needs to be addressed.

It was through the door of PMS that I first learned about natural hormones nearly twenty years ago. Prior to that time I had been working at a high-risk pregnancy facility at the University of California at Los Angeles and had set my sights on a career in research. When the program sud-

TYPICAL SYMPTOMS OF PMS

Physical

- Water retention: "I feel like I am going through labor."
- Breast tenderness: "They are hot, tender, and painful."
- Fatigue: "I just want to lie down and sleep."

Emotional

- Mood swings: "A demon enters my mind and controls me."
- Depression: "Everything seems dark and gloomy."
- Anxiety: "I feel very fragile and afraid."
- Irritability: "When I feel this way, I can't stand the people around me."
- Craving for sweets: "I never thought that I would ever crave Twinkies."
- Craving for chocolate: "It's like being thirsty for water in the desert."

denly closed, I was out of grant money and out of a job. I was in a new city with a wife and three young children. I didn't have many contacts outside the confines of the research community. I now had to go out and find work.

Because my English was lacking at the time, it wasn't easy. But I gradually managed to find work as a staff gynecologist at a number of clinics around Southern California.

This was a unique experience. I saw people with widely differing views on the nature of healing and health care. I served as the medical doctor for midwives and drugless practitioners. I saw patients in one clinic headed by brilliant physicians affiliated with the Scientology movement. They used medical drugs only minimally and no mind-altering medication at all. I also treated many Hare Krishna followers and devotees of a famous spiritual guru.

I learned a great deal about methods I had never encountered in medical school. And I also learned a great deal about patient individuality.

In 1981 I attended a series of lectures by Guy Abraham, M.D., a former professor of gynecology at UCLA who had developed a nutritional approach to PMS. His ideas opened my eyes to a whole new world of nutritional healing potential that I had never been taught in medical school—neither in Israel, in Europe, nor in the United States.

I then learned about the work of Katharina Dalton, the London physician who started the first PMS clinic in the world in 1953. Dalton pioneered the effectiveness of natural progesterone therapy.

Inspired by these new ideas, I opened a clinic in Los Angeles in 1982 specializing in PMS treatment with nutrition and progesterone. The results were excellent. I was helping many women who had failed to improve with "standard treatments."

At that time, PMS symptoms were largely ignored or dismissed by the medical establishment. Patients often complained to me about doctors who told them "it was all in their heads." Fortunately, these views have changed and come full circle. Nowadays, women are prescribed a whole cocktail of drugs for PMS symptoms, including Prozac and Zoloft for depression, Ativan, Xanax, and Valium for relaxation, and sleeping pills if they can't sleep.

Before discussing the progesterone approach, let me take a minute to share with you some important information regarding nutrition and PMS. If you choose to follow any of these suggestions, give yourself up to three months to see results. Your patience will be rewarded.

- Cut down on empty calories, that is, junk foods containing a lot of sugar.
- Cut down on any form of hydrogenated fats in your diet. Hydrogenated fats, typically found in processed foods, are used to extend the shelf life of products. These substances, called "trans fats," displace essential fats in the membranes of cells and interfere with critical membrane functions.
- Cut down on your intake of calcium. That's right. Cut down. I believe, as do many nutritionally oriented physicians, that women are overloading on calcium and not getting enough magnesium. Indeed, surveys repeatedly show that 75 percent of the population is deficient in magnesium.

Yes, we all need calcium for healthy bones, but you won't achieve good bone health without adequate magnesium. Magnesium increases bone elasticity. A deficiency can contribute to osteoporosis.

Moreover, magnesium is often the nutritional missing link to menstrual wellness. Some studies have linked PMS to magnesium deficiency alone, or in combination with excess calcium.

According to Mildred Seelig, Ph.D., author of a major medical textbook on the magnesium-disease connection and an adjunct professor of family and preventive medicine at Emory University in Atlanta, the widespread nature of magnesium deficiency is a serious yet unheralded cause of death and suffering.

The mineral is a major partner in more than three hundred enzymatic reactions in the body, including the generation of cellular energy and muscle relaxation, and the synthesis of fat, protein, and nucleic acids. Deficiency is involved in a wide range of symptoms, premenstrual difficulties among them, but also life-threatening convulsions, arrhythmias, and heart attacks.

We tend not to eat enough of the foods that are rich in magnesium, such as green vegetables, nuts, soy, and whole grains. Our unfortunate preference for processed foods guarantees a low magnesium intake and all the health risks related to deficiency. The refining of whole grains eliminates most of the magnesium content. For example, the processing of whole wheat to white flour causes a magnesium loss of 82 percent.

The obsession with calcium in our society appears to be a major contributor to magnesium depletion. High intake of calcium interferes with magnesium absorption. In other words it makes an already existing deficiency worse.

So we need to hear more than just the calcium message. We need to start hearing the magnesium message.

One reason why so many women with PMS crave chocolate is because most of them are magnesium deficient. Chocolate contains a high concentration of magnesium. So maybe at some primordial level, while your body is crying for magnesium, you instinctively reach for something that addresses the need and the stress at the same time. Scientists, by the way, have found that chemicals in chocolate are attracted to the same brain receptor system targeted by marijuana. There may be a genuine mood elevation effect involved besides the immediate gratification of the taste buds. Medicating yourself with chocolate has its downsides though. Chocolate is also high in refined sugar, which can cause problems with your blood sugar levels and exacerbate PMS.

On page 153 is a chart with a daily nutritional supplementation program I have developed over the years that can significantly decrease and often even prevent many PMS problems. I find it improves symptoms in about three-quarters of my PMS patients. You can purchase these supplements at a health food store.

Natural Progesterone for PMS

Start progesterone at day fifteen, or three days before the onset of symptoms. As long as you experience PMS symptoms, you aren't taking enough progesterone.

Sublingual drops work the best because of the constant need to adjust the dosage. Refer to my general guidelines for administering drops in chapter 13.

Sublingual drops. Start with a low dose. You don't want to create responses related to excess progesterone. Take four to eight drops in the evening and two to six in the morning. Adjust your level according to your symptoms.

I suggest keeping the bottle of progesterone handy throughout the day. Use more drops as needed if you have only partial relief. That may become necessary, as symptoms intensify closer to the beginning of your next period. Be aware that the intensity often fluctuates from month to month.

Stop the sublingual drops at day twenty-eight when the period arrives.

About a third of my PMS patients have symptoms that extend into their period. For these women, I recommend continuing with the progesterone at a dosage equal to half of what they take just prior to the onset of menstruation. For instance, if they were taking sixteen drops at night and twelve in the morning, they would continue with eight at night and six in the morning during their period. They slowly decrease the amount and stop the drops at the end of the period.

ANTI-PMS SUPPLEMENT PROGRAM

Magnesium Glycinate

This form of magnesium provides superb absorption. Magnesium in excess can cause a laxative or drowsiness effect. Try to take as much as you can to achieve two soft bowel movements a day but without experiencing a strong, sedative effect.

I use a glycinate product made by Metagenics. In general, I suggest one to four 200-milligram capsules twice a day. Use as much as is tolerable. If you can't find this product, look for magnesium aspartate in your health food store.

Gamma-Linoleic Acid (GLA)

Take 400 milligrams daily. This fatty acid is the active ingredient in evening primrose oil.

B Complex

Take 100 milligrams daily.

Vitamin B$_6$

Take 50 to 600 milligrams in divided doses over the day. Start low. Increase as needed.

You may recall a negative study on B$_6$ conducted in the 1980s that got a lot of media attention. It appeared to link doses over 750 milligrams to nervous system damage. Subsequent research has clarified the issue. The actual problem was a relative deficiency of vitamin B$_2$ that developed when very high doses (up to 2,000 milligrams) of B$_6$ were taken alone. Anytime you take a large amount of one of the B vitamins, you should always take a full-range B complex vitamin as well. This prevents the development of a deficiency and imbalance among the other B vitamins. I have recommended high doses of B$_6$ and B complex to many patients without any problem. B$_6$ is very useful for reducing fluid retention.

An Herbal Diuretic

Available in health food stores. Follow label instructions.

Capsules: For the first three or four cycles, take 25- or 50-milligram potency pills. This allows you to easily find the best individual level and adjust upward or downward according to your needs.

Start with 50 milligrams at night and 25 or 50 milligrams with breakfast or lunch. Increase the dosage as long as you have symptoms. If you take too much you will develop signs of excess. Reduce the amount if that happens.

Creams: I recommend this form only for mild PMS or if a patient develops a paradoxical response to progesterone, even if the amount of progesterone is small.

As I explained earlier, the paradoxical response refers to the few women for whom a slight amount of extra progesterone can cause signs of excess. In these situations, I prescribe a very weak cream—½ to 1 percent strength. The potency can be slowly increased to tolerance level, however I find that most will react even to the OTC creams at 1.5 or 3 percent strength.

In my experience, only individuals with very mild PMS respond positively to creams. Most women with more severe PMS do not even respond to the 10 percent cream.

Vaginal suppositories: This was the original method of replacement when natural progesterone first became available to practitioners in the early 1980s. I prescribed suppositories exclusively until other forms were developed a decade later. Many practitioners still prescribe only suppositories. They may not be aware of the newer options.

The doses I recommend in order to achieve benefits are relatively high, namely suppositories at 200- to 400-milligram strength administered three or four times a day.

This method concentrates the hormone in the pelvic area. Here, that's a drawback because PMS is a systemic disorder.

One advantage of this method, however, is that it rarely causes a paradoxical effect and you can use much higher doses of progesterone.

Monitoring Your Intake

Your optimum level is what you need to experience relief of symptoms without side effects of excess progesterone.

Women on Birth Control Pills

If you take the pill, you should know what's in it. You have chemicalized estrogen plus a progestin. It contains no progesterone.

Most of the progestins in the pill initially involved a breed of drug derived from male testosterone. Research on this substance relates mostly to decreasing the side effects associated with a male hormone, such as acne or oily skin, and to addressing the detrimental effect of progestins on cholesterol.

Many millions of women count on birth control pills. I believe that the manufacturers have a great responsibility to provide a safe product. Any new progestins brought to market should first be thoroughly tested for their effects on the coronary arteries and breast tissue. They should ensure that as a result of taking these drugs for twenty or thirty years, women do not increase the risk of breast cancer and coronary artery constriction. If these companies don't want to use natural progesterone as part of the birth control pill, they should surely see to it that their patented, chemicalized hormonal substitutes give to women the same bone and cancer protection.

In the early 1990s, Depo-Provera was officially approved in the United States as an injectible contraceptive after two decades of concern and debate about its safety. It is advertised as more effective and convenient than the pill. With this method, a woman receives an injection every three months.

In my opinion, any form of Provera—whether delivered via pill or injection—is suspect. This drug is known to create chaos in the rhythm of the cycle. Sometimes it takes more than a year after stopping the injections before regularity returns. There are concerns also about long-term negative effects on the eyes and bone mineral density.

Natural Progesterone for Women Taking the Birth Control Pill

I routinely tell my younger patients about the benefits of progesterone. Any form of natural progesterone they would be willing to take is fine with me. I urge them to at least apply a topical cream to the breasts.

Most of the time, however, the prospect of an increased risk of disease many years away isn't a strong enough selling point to motivate them. Younger women are less likely to follow a hormonal replacement program. For those who have the interest, any of the following methods are helpful:

Creams/gels: Apply a 10 percent potency cream to the body and breasts at least once daily, and preferably twice.

Many times I suggest the over-the-counter 3 percent cream because I know that younger patients are simply going to be less compliant. They tend to feel no compelling reason to take a prescriptive cream, so they opt for the convenience of the OTC product.

Let me just say that there is really no evidence that the low-potency cream offers the same protection as the higher strength cream. Moreover, I know for sure that any cream applied solely to the breasts will not yield the systemic benefits of progesterone capsules or sublingual drops. So apply to the body as well, following the general guidelines for using creams.

Capsules: Take 100 milligrams before sleep and 50 milligrams at breakfast or lunch. Apply the cream to the breasts.

BETTER CONTRACEPTIVES?

I am not a pharmaceutical researcher, but I would like to suggest the two following ideas as possible improvements to the chemicalized contraceptives available to women today.

The Dream Pill

My idea of a "dream pill" excludes progestin. Such a pill would retain the aggressive estrogen component to suppress ovulation. But it would include estriol, the very protective estrogen compound, for balance. The early use of contraceptives by very young women has been shown to increase the risk of breast cancer. A pill with estriol could affect cellular activity in a positive way and prevent or delay cancer.

I would also include progesterone for all its many benefits. It might not be possible to include both these elements in one pill. That's mainly because progesterone needs to be taken twice a day. But if you had to take two pills and they reduced the risk of breast cancer, I don't think that's too much to ask.

Dream Cream?

I have noticed among young patients that when they use progesterone cream or gel vaginally they achieve the same contraceptive effect as the pill but without any side effects.

The cream appears to prevent pregnancy by decreasing the endometrial lining of the uterus where implantation of the fertilized egg takes place. Furthermore, the daily use of the cream throughout the whole month could eliminate the production of cervical mucus, another key element in conception.

If my observation is correct, the implications are powerful. Imagine a natural contraceptive hormonal cream with no short- or long-term side effects.

No weight gain. No acne. No mood changes. No water retention. No headaches.

I don't have enough information to say this is a proven method of birth control. And I am not recommending that anyone use it for that.

I would like to see the pharmaceutical companies put some research into this. If indeed it is effective, compliance and usage—not to mention sales— could be astronomical. Why not give women a great natural contraceptive option instead of just drugs?

One obstacle that would have to be solved is the potential for abnormal bleeding when progesterone is used vaginally on a daily basis.

Sublingual drops. Take eight to twelve drops before sleep and four to six in the morning. Rub a few drops on the breasts once a day.

Women with Cystic (Lumpy) Breasts

"My breasts are full of lumps."

"I can't stand my breasts . . . they are painful and cystic."

"I can't examine my breasts anymore because they are so full of lumps and fibrous tissue."

There isn't a day in my practice that I don't hear comments like this. Probably a third of my new patients express concern. Most of the time the problem relates to what we call benign cystic breast disease.

The frequency with which patients bring this situation to my attention is a constant reminder of the widespread fear of breast cancer.

Let me set the record straight:

First, there is no connection between the common lumps and breast cancer, as long as a woman is not in estrogen dominance.

The lumps are typically a call for progesterone. Estrogen promotes the growth and proliferation of breast cells. An excess of estrogen that is not balanced by progesterone can result in greater breast cell growth, which you experience as lumps.

If the development of lumps occurs only premenstrually, follow my guidelines in the previous section on PMS.

If the lumps are not associated with your cycle, the following program will generally reduce or eliminate the problem:

- **10 percent progesterone gel (prescription item).** Apply the gel once or twice a day to your breasts. There is no need to apply the gel to the nipples, but be sure to cover the upper extremities of the breasts toward the armpits. The breast tissue just below the armpits contains many glandular cells.
- **Cut out caffeine.** Caffeine contributes to cystic breasts. Elimination of caffeine products (coffee, tea, and soft drinks) can make a big difference.
- **Natural vitamin E (mixed gamma and alpha tocopherols).** Buy it in a health food store. Take 400 international units (IUs) twice daily. Soft gel capsules with vitamin E are available in 400 IU strength.

Women with Infertility Concerns

One of the most common reasons for infertility is corpus luteum insufficiency, which is also the cause of abnormal bleeding. The body lacks adequate progesterone.

For years, infertility doctors have used progesterone injections, capsules, or vaginal suppositories. They haven't used Provera or other progestins. And why not? Because they are aware of the problems with progestins, and especially Provera, and the possibility that these drugs could increase the incidence of birth defects.

Lately, however, many of these physicians have been influenced by new reports on the use of Crinone, the vaginal progesterone cream, in the treatment of infertility. I have a problem with this limited approach. It steers the benefits of progesterone to the uterus and leaves the rest of the body less protected. Remember that the vaginal route of progesterone replacement concentrates the hormone in the pelvic cavity.

I prefer a whole body approach. I want progesterone's "extended protection warranty" to benefit the breasts as well. Research shows that women with lower progesterone have a higher incidence of cancer. So I routinely suggest to my patients that they use a systemic form of progesterone—capsules or sublingual drops.

There's another problem here. Many women undergoing fertility treatment are prescribed medications that increase their estrogen level. This also heightens the threat of estrogen dominance, which the vaginal progesterone replacement route is inadequate to address. In these situations, I would urge you to ask your infertility doctor about taking some form of systemic progesterone. The progesterone should be added following ovulation.

Progesterone and Postpartum Depression

During my medical career I have delivered thousands of babies. I have learned to observe brand-new mothers very closely and watch for even the slightest signs of depression. Even the lack of smiling tells me that something may be wrong. Postpartum depression can be very serious and devastating to both the new mother and the family. It needs to be nipped right in the bud.

I don't agree that this condition is normal. It is very abnormal. Giving birth should be a peak and joyous time in a woman's life.

How can it happen? Recent research shows that the towering hormonal levels during pregnancy come crashing down after childbirth. In a few days, a woman's level of progesterone falls to nearly zero. During pregnancy it is significantly higher than normal. The subsequent crash gives us the clue to the solution.

At the first sign of depression or any lack of joy, while the new mother is still in the hospital, I strongly recommend the use of progesterone. If she does not think she needs it, or doesn't feel she is even slightly depressed, I advise her and her husband to be watchful for any developing signs.

If she agrees to the progesterone treatment, I inject 200 milligrams of the hormone daily for as long as she stays in the hospital. Progesterone injectibles are available in all hospitals.

Many times, women who are seriously depressed, dysfunctional, and even suicidal are returned to normalcy within eight to twelve hours after the injection. I have seen many miraculous transformations. And if they are not miraculous, women at least go from being dysfunctional to functional and slowly improve.

I also prescribe a 0.1-milligram estrogen patch (Vivelle-Dot, or other similar products that are available). The reason for this is that estrogen levels also drop drastically after childbirth. When the patient returns home, I switch her to one of the Tri-Est formulas.

This simple approach, plus a follow-up home program, has resolved more than 90 percent of postpartum cases I have seen. In twenty years of obstetrical experience, only a few patients have needed aggressive psychiatric intervention.

One important fact to remember is this: the earlier you react to signs of depression, and begin this approach, the better you are able to prevent it from becoming serious.

At home, I recommend the following routine:

- **Progesterone.** Take 100 to 150 milligrams at bedtime and 50 to 200 milligrams in the morning, or 10 percent gel A.M. and P.M. In these situations, symptoms of excess progesterone, such as dizziness, are extremely rare.

    Nevertheless, in recognition of a woman's weakened physical state, it is prudent to watch for any such sign.

    Some women will also need a periodic progesterone injection—once every three to ten days for a few months—to keep them even.
- **Estrogen.** Take 1 gram of the basic Tri-Est gel or a 2.25-milligram Tri-Est capsule twice daily.

In severe cases, I also add the following:

- **St. John's wort.** Take one capsule of the standard extract three times daily. A rare side effect from taking this herb is photosensitivity.
- **5-HTP (5-hydroxy L-tryptophan).** Take 100 to 150 milligrams of this natural serotonin enhancer, at bedtime, plus 50 milligrams at breakfast and lunch. In a month's time, you may increase the breakfast and lunch dosage to 100 milligrams, if needed. Serotonin is a brain chemical. Low levels are

associated with depression. 5-HTP may generate, in a natural way, the same benefits of Prozac and other antidepressant medications. Too much 5-HTP can make you sleepy or bring on loose bowels. If this occurs, decrease the quantity or take it with food.

Once I treated a nurse who had developed postpartum depression. Her pediatrician had referred her to me.

It turned out that the nurse worked for one of the most recognized psychiatric experts on the subject of pharmaceutical treatment of postpartum depression. The psychiatrist had prescribed an antidepressant drug called a selective serotonin reuptake inhibitor (SSRI). This is a relatively new and important type of drug for depression and mood disorders. Current research with these drugs on pregnancy and breast-feeding is extremely limited. As yet there is no clear indication they are without risk to the fetus or newborn. For this reason the pediatrician suggested the nurse stop breast-feeding if she took the drug.

I understand the seriousness of postpartum depression and I believe that correcting such depression even takes priority over breast-feeding. But I also believe that progesterone is a safer way to go most of the time.

The nurse responded rapidly and positively to a single injection. Her response was similar to many I have witnessed in the same situation. Often within four to twelve hours there is a dramatic change.

The following day I received a call from the nurse's boss, the postpartum depression expert.

"What did you give her?" she demanded in a hostile voice.

"I gave her progesterone," I said.

"I reviewed all the medical literature and progesterone doesn't work," she screamed.

"Well, what do you want me to say?" I said. "I gave her progesterone and nothing else."

That effectively ended the conservation.

This is an example to me of the close-mindedness of many medical professionals to the possibility that there are other methods besides drugs.

Other physicians have sometimes told me that the results I am getting with natural hormones are probably just placebo effects. Well, I doubt if a placebo effect can turn a woman in the throes of deep postpartum depression into a happy, functional new mother. A placebo effect, in my understanding, means that the body decides to heal itself. Maybe indeed this is what we do when we give the body the natural hormone is it missing. And maybe this is just the right and most effective thing to do, instead of a drug that often causes new problems besides suppressing the symptoms of the old problem.

If a woman experiences postpartum depression once, she is likely to have it again after her second childbirth. To prevent this, the following program of progesterone intramuscular injections can be applied:

- 100 to 200 milligrams once a week, starting at the thirty-fifth week of pregnancy.
- The same dosage immediately after delivery and every day while in the hospital.
- The same dosage once a week for ten weeks, or as needed.

This program was developed by Katharina Dalton, the pioneering British physician who first used natural progesterone. It is successful most of the time.

PART FOUR

Building on the Basics: Using Other Natural Hormones to Stay Younger, More Vital, and Healthier

Testosterone

Testosterone at a Glance

Testosterone is not just "a man thing." Female ovaries produce far less than men do, but that little bit goes a long way.

Research, along with clinical experience, shows that testosterone in a woman contributes to the following:

- Stamina. "My endurance is much greater."
- Healthy and stronger muscles. "I have more strength in my arms."
- Lean body mass and less body fat. "I like my new lean cut."
- Stronger bones.
- A feeling of security, positivity, and stability. "I just feel safer."
- Increased libido, orgasmic power, and enhanced emotional aspect of sexuality. "I feel like a college kid again."
- Higher nitric oxide, a naturally occurring substance that helps keep blood vessels dilated.
- Protection against plaque in the blood vessels.
- Improved balance and hand-to-eye coordination. "I have more balance in my yoga class."

Like so many of the other hormones, the testosterone level peaks around the age of twenty-five and then slowly declines. The level of testosterone is subject to quite typical fluctuations in the body. It is higher during the day and around the time of ovulation.

Signs of Testosterone Deficiency

- Flabbiness and muscular weakness. The decrease of muscle tone is typically seen in sagging upper arms and cheeks. Women often tell me, "I dislike my flabby arms. What can I do about it?"
- Loss of hair: "I thought that only men lose their hair."
- Lack of energy and stamina: "I drag through my aerobics class."
- Loss of coordination and balance: "I seem to fall more frequently when I ski."
- Loss of sense of security: "I don't feel safe."
- Indecisiveness: "I just can't seem to make up my mind about anything."
- Decreased sex drive: "I don't care."
- Poor body image: "I don't like my body."
- Decreased armpit, pubic, and body hair: "What does it mean that I'm losing my hair?"

Proper testosterone replacement reverses these situations. Frequently, tall, thin, flat-chested younger women who are low in estrogen tend also to be low in testosterone. Replacement helps them as well.

Testosterone Is a Prescription Item

You will need a doctor's prescription to obtain testosterone. Ask your physician to call or fax a compounding pharmacy (see Appendix A) to order the hormone for you.

Testosterone is available in capsules, gels, creams, and sublingual drops.

If you wish to combine testosterone with other hormones, refer to my guidelines in chapter 22.

In order to assure optimum results with testosterone replacement, be sure your diet or supplement program contains adequate zinc and vitamin A.

Who Should Take Testosterone

"Women have testosterone?"

"I need testosterone?"

I've heard these remarks from hundreds of surprised patients over the years whenever I've told them that not only do they have testosterone, but that they would greatly benefit from taking it.

"Please don't worry," I've told them, "you won't become hairy or bald like me. It will do you a lot of good."

On a first visit to my office, when I do a physical examination, I analyze a patient for certain estrogen qualities and similarly for their androgenicity. This term refers to male hormone influences in the body.

I assess hair distribution and musculature. The more muscle and hair a woman has the more testosterone activity in the body. The two often go hand in hand. Obviously, if a woman is a bodybuilder, you cannot assess her muscle mass as a physiological indicator of her testosterone level.

In general, more musculature, but little hair distribution over the body, indicates reduced 5-alpha reductase ability. This refers to the enzyme that converts testosterone into dihydrotestosterone, a closely related substance that promotes the growth of body hair. More musculature and little hair also indicates a high "aromatization" ability, a term used to describe a cellular process in which testosterone converts to estrogen.

Obviously, men have a much greater ability to convert testosterone to dihydrotestosterone and a lesser ability for the estrogen conversion. Yet if we see a male with a lot of hair on his head and none on the body, he converts some testosterone also into estrogen. That is regarded as a sign of increased risk for prostate cancer.

When I consider the androgenicity of a woman during the initial office visit, I am trying to assess her hormonal balance when she was younger.

The major research on testosterone in women relates to its effect on the sexual response. The whole essence of sexuality—from self-image as a sexual being to sexual performance—is enhanced. But researchers at Canada's McGill University have determined that increased sexual motivation develops only when women take doses that are relatively high.

I look at testosterone replacement in a broader context. I see it as a major benefactor for women. *Its effects are very central to strength, vitality, and emotions.*

The medical community is starting to recognize the benefits of testosterone for women. As expected, it uses chemicalized versions of the hormone, particularly methyltestosterone. This drug provides some of the benefits of testosterone but is known to be toxic to the liver.

Here is another case where advancements in chemistry have provided the technology to reproduce the exact replica of human testosterone from plants. Yet for the medical community, the exact replica of our own testosterone is apparently not good enough.

If the health of patients is the paramount objective in medical research, why not do research on the readily available identical natural substance instead of a potentially harmful drug? If pharmaceutical companies won't do it, why doesn't the government fund such research?

In good conscience I cannot prescribe a drug to a patient that will damage her liver when I can use a natural hormone product identical to what she has in her body.

Testosterone for Younger Women

The benefits from supplementation are many—at any age. I have seen testosterone help women in their teens and early twenties. Many younger women, in fact, show signs of deficiency simply because their bodies produce smaller amounts of the hormone.

Testosterone can help develop more stamina, stronger muscles, and feelings of strength and security. It reduces fat and anxiety.

Testosterone at Perimenopause

By the time a woman reaches thirty-five there is a substantial decline in testosterone. The rate of decline, of course, varies.

With the decline, bone strength and cardiovascular protection are reduced. Physically, you may notice a decrease in the amount of pubic and armpit hair. You may also start seeing some of the emotional and sexual signs of testosterone deficiency.

There is also a major vanity impact. When a women looks in the mirror and notices that her skin isn't as tight as it used to be, that's a symptom of declining testosterone. Skin tone suffers as the muscles beneath lose their firmness, strength, and size.

Testosterone in Menopause

Even though the body's production of testosterone falls with age, the relative rate of estrogen loss is much steeper than testosterone. This sets up an interesting phenomenon. As a woman ages, she might begin showing signs of testosterone excess, such as hair on the face and loss of head and body hair.

How can this happen? Please refer back to chapter 5, where I discussed the sex hormone–binding globulin (SHBG). You will remember this as the protein made in the liver that accompanies hormones around the body. It is part of the wondrous system of the body's inner intelligence. SHBG governs the availability of hormones for use by the cells. The higher the level of estrogen, the greater the binding effect of SHBG on estrogen as well as other hormones, including testosterone. So now in menopause, with the estrogen level dropping dramatically, the SHBG level drops as well, releasing more of the remaining testosterone in the body to be available to testosterone-sensitive cells.

Interestingly, testosterone replacement in men can reduce SHBG and enhance the body's ability to use other hormones. It does not have the same effect for women.

In aging men, testosterone plays a major role in cardiovascular and antidiabetic protection. The relatively smaller amount of testosterone in the female body suggests that such protection may be minor.

Nevertheless, menopausal women have a great deal to gain from testosterone. Better balance and hand-to-eye coordination is one important benefit. We hear much about older women falling and fracturing bones. Researchers have found that men have fewer fractures from falls than women. One reason is the higher testosterone level. Men tend to fall less. When they do fall they have superior hand-to-eye coordination, which allows them to more effectively break the impact. Proper supplementation with testosterone might reduce the incidence of serious injuries that occur when older women fall. Moreover, a higher level of testosterone also helps to build stronger bones.

For a woman who has had her ovaries removed, I believe that testosterone should be part of her hormonal replacement therapy.

Before Starting Testosterone

Your physician should test your blood level for two values: total testosterone and free testosterone. The normal range of total testosterone is typically between 30 to 80 ng/dl. A woman with little muscle and body hair might have a level in the 20 to 40 ng/dl range. A more muscular and hairy woman will probably be up in the 75 to 100 range.

As I have indicated, the availability of testosterone in your body is directly governed by the presence of the sex hormone–binding globulin. Indirectly, it is also governed by estrogen. A naturally high estrogen level, or estrogen replacement therapy by mouth, or large doses of estrogen sublingual drops, all translate to an increase in SHBG. That means more testosterone is bound up. The actual level of the available (free) testosterone is reduced. For this reason, you want to have your level of free testosterone checked as well.

The ability of SHBG to bind testosterone is the mechanism behind the birth control pill's antiacne benefit. Excessive testosterone can cause oily skin and acne formation. The aggressive estrogens in the pill increase SHBG. This, in turn, decreases the amount of free testosterone, resulting in reduced acne and possibly also less hair growth.

Keep in mind though that testosterone has many important benefits for the woman taking the birth control pill. It builds bone, muscle, and skin tissue. It affects stamina, sexuality, and the sense of security. These influences are reduced when SHBG is high.

How to Take Testosterone

A good indicator for a starting dose of testosterone is the amount of body hair and musculature. Start low if you have comparatively little hair and muscle development. Start low also if you have more than average hair and more ample muscle development, but a testosterone level over 40 ng/dl. The same woman, with a low testosterone level, under 20 ng/dl, should start higher. You will find my dosage recommendations for each specific form of testosterone in the following sections of the chapter.

Increase your dosage gradually. There is a direct dosage relationship to benefits and side effects. The more you take the greater the potential benefits. The more you take the greater the potential for side effects as well. Some individuals may not tolerate the needed dosage in order to reach their goal. Your body will tell you, usually within two to six weeks, if you're taking too much. Be on the lookout for the signs.

Side effects are usually associated with a significantly elevated blood level of testosterone. Yet not everyone with an elevated level experiences signs of excess.

Signs of Excess Testosterone

- Aggressiveness. "My husband complains that I am too pushy."
- Bossiness. "My employees say I'm too tough on them."
- Oily skin. "My skin seems to ooze with oil."
- Acne, not just limited to the face. Could be the back, sides, and face: "Where are these pimples coming from?"
- When using creams/gels, hair might appear at the site where the preparation is applied to the body. "I see hair growing, and it bothers me."
- Loss of head hair, along with the growth of facial hair: "It seems like the hair I'm losing on the top of my head is growing back on my chin." (Women who take too much, and yet do not show other typical signs, may develop very mild hair growth on the face after two or three months.)

Applying Testosterone Gel

This is the best way to go in most cases. Gel offers the most flexibility in covering both systemic and localized goals.

I start most women with 0.2 to 0.4 percent gel (see strength of gel below). The quantity of gel can be increased by 50 percent every four weeks. Begin with 1 gram (a quarter teaspoon) in the morning. Rub it onto the following three areas of the body:

1. Either the right or left inner thigh. This application benefits the whole body, including the bones, muscles, cardiovascular system, and the emotions.
2. The perineum, the nonhairy area between the vagina and the rectum. The gel is absorbed through the skin and distributes testosterone throughout the pelvic cavity. This serves to strengthen and restore the bladder muscle, the sexual organs and pelvic muscles above.
3. The small labia. This targets the vagina more precisely.

If any side effects are encountered, stop for a week. Then start reapplying the gel at half the previous quantity you used. If you see new signs of excess developing, or there is no relief from the previous signs, stop the gel once again. This time wait until all the signs have vanished and restart at half the amount your were previously using.

I generally start with the lower potency (0.2 percent) if a woman has a considerable amount of body hair and an average blood level of total testosterone. If she has a low blood level, I start higher. Her body probably produced a higher level when she was younger. The presence of more hair means that your body converts testosterone more readily into dihydrotestosterone, which in turn promotes more hair growth. I also start lower if a person has a relatively higher blood level of testosterone.

A low blood level, combined with a small degree of body hair, means that you don't readily convert testosterone to dihydrotestosterone. I would start with a low dose because the body is not accustomed to a high dose of testosterone.

My patients tell me that the once-a-day morning dose usually suffices to reduce depression and anxiousness while generating a feeling of positivity, security, confidence, and sexuality throughout the day.

Enhancing Your Orgasmic Response

If you are interested in enhancing your orgasmic response, you might try the following technique fifteen minutes to a half hour before sexual activity:

Stimulate the clitoris for one or two minutes in order to enhance blood flow engorgement. Then apply a small amount of gel to the clitoris. Experiment to learn what works best for you. Six or seven out of ten patients who try this technique tell me they experience increased sexual performance. They report the following benefits:

- Stronger orgasm
- Multiple orgasms
- More sexual gratification.

At least 20 percent of sexually active women do not achieve a vaginal orgasm. They experience a feeling of orgasm only through clitoral stimulation. With the use of the gel, about a third of such women will reach a full and pleasurable vaginal climax. For some of my patients, testosterone replacement enables them to achieve a full orgasm for the first time.

The enhancement of the sexual benefit usually requires a higher quantity of gel. But a high amount on a daily basis might generate signs of testosterone excess. Here are two ways to avoid it:

1. Use a higher dose every other day.
2. Use a high dose and then stop for two or three days.

The strategy depends on how much you increase in order to achieve your immediate goal. The more you increase, the longer the delay before you resume taking it again.

Recently I have started prescribing dihydrotestosterone gel to patients desiring even greater sexual pleasure. The gel is applied to the clitoris before sex. This close cousin to testosterone appears to generate more intense gratification. However, it is more expensive and with daily use might cause both unwanted hair growth and hair loss.

There is no correlation between the testosterone blood level and sexual performance in a woman. Some individuals have a very high level of testosterone and little sexual desire. Others with a low level could have nymphomaniac tendencies. Each person is individual. And no one can tell you precisely what is your ideal dosage based on a blood level. The blood test, however, provides a baseline for treatment.

Strength of Gel

Each gram of the basic gel I prescribe contains from 0.05 to 0.6 percent testosterone. One gram is equal to a quarter of a teaspoon. Most women will develop side effects with a gel stronger than 0.6 percent.

Taking Capsules

I usually start a patient with 2.5 milligrams twice a day with meals.

Some women experience adequate daylong benefits after taking testosterone once a day in the morning. Others feel they need it twice a day.

If you are interested in enhancing your sexual performance, I suggest taking the second dose about two hours before intercourse.

Strength of Capsules

Capsules are available in 0.5- to 5-milligram strength.

Taking Sublingual Drops

I usually start with two drops a day, taken in the morning. Remember I am talking about drops, and not dropperfuls. The dosage can be increased every two to four weeks. The maximum dose a patient ever took without developing side effects was eight drops twice daily.

Stop the drops at the first signs of excess. When the signs disappear, you can resume the drops again. Symptoms usually take a few weeks to clear up. Resume at a level 25 percent less than what you took previously.

For enhanced sexual pleasure, I suggest administering one drop and rubbing it on the clitoris about a half hour to forty-five minutes before sex. The absorption rate of the testosterone drops may be slightly less effective than the gel.

Strength of Sublingual Drops

Each drop contains 1 milligram of testosterone.

Monitoring Your Intake with Your Physician

The most important factor in monitoring testosterone is how you feel. You want to achieve your goals without the appearance of side effects.

Here are three examples:

1. You experience side effects and your blood level shows just a moderately higher amount of testosterone. You are taking too much. Stop until the side effects diminish. Restart with one-third less.
2. You achieve significant benefits, such as elimination of depression, enhanced sexuality, weight loss, improved muscle growth, and a greater sense of security. You have no signs of testosterone excess, but your blood level is higher than "normal." As long as you have no signs of excess, and you are happy with the results, you have no reason to reduce your dosage. But if you experience the most minimal side effects, cut down a notch. Such a sign could be people saying you are getting bossy.
3. Some women don't seem to mind the side effects in order to reach their goal. They don't mind the trade-off. I discourage this approach. You must listen to your body.

Measuring your testosterone blood level is critical, and a useful tool in helping to assess your response.

Once you have been taking testosterone for about three months, you should recheck your blood level. The blood draw should be about six to eight hours after taking the hormone. If, for convenience sake, you can only do the blood draw earlier in the day, remember that the level will be higher. For instance, a blood draw three hours after you take the hormone will show a peak level that will be significantly higher than the level found later in the day. Your real average level is about 30 to 40 percent below the peak.

Many patients enjoy the sense of strength and empowerment that comes with testosterone but tend not to notice the emotional or personality changes it causes when taken in excess. Aggressiveness, overconfidence, and bossiness are typical signs of too much testosterone.

When I see test results with relatively high blood levels, I ask patients if their husbands, children, lovers, or colleagues are complaining.

Yes, they often say, the people in their lives have commented that they've become domineering or pushy.

Women usually become concerned only when their looks are affected, for instance, when they notice unwanted hair growth, oily skin, or acne. Some individuals don't even care about that as long as they are getting the benefits.

Whenever any signs of excess testosterone develop—either at the physical or personality level—the body is telling you to take less. And that's what I tell my patients to do.

Three Testosterone Stories

Let me share several cases that will give you an insight on the use of testosterone.

CHANTALE'S STORY

Chantale roared into my office, pounded her right fist on my desk, and announced: "I feel great. This testosterone is fabulous."

"Are you using the drops as I recommended?" I asked.

"Oh yes, I use only one," she answered.

"One what? One drop or one dropperful?"

"Well, I just put the dropper in and fill it one time."

"Is anybody complaining about your personality?" I asked.

"Oh, people are complaining all the time," she said. "They liked me better when I was quiet, shy, and docile. Right now I feel free and strong for the first time in my life."

Chantale was obviously taking too much testosterone. I did a blood draw and found her level twice as high as normal. Yet, besides turning from a mouse into a lion, she experienced no other significant sign of excess testosterone. Her skin had previously been very dry. Now it was slightly oily. She liked it that way. She noticed some slight regrowth of pubic and armpit hair.

In short, Chantale was happy. I did convince her, however, to take a reduced amount of testosterone. She had too many signs of excess, and her blood level was too high.

SUZANNE'S STORY

By nature, this forty-year-old lawyer was a hardworking yet basically shy person. During an office visit she complained of lack of stamina and sex drive.

I suggested that testosterone could energize her private and professional life. At my recommendation she started using testosterone gel. She soon became an expert.

During a subsequent office visit she told me she doubles her dosage on court appearance days.

"The testosterone increases my confidence, assertiveness, and effectiveness," Suzanne said.

She would also use more than normal on days when she had office meetings or had to see clients. On days of research and writing, she would use less, or none at all.

On the weekends, she generally wouldn't use testosterone unless she was having sex. Then she would apply the gel a half hour before intercourse.

"My sex drive and pleasure have benefited enormously," Suzanne told me.

Here is a good example of mastering the use of testosterone to serve your daily needs without creating signs of excess. Many women in my practice have done the same.

RITA'S STORY

Rita is an avid surfer. She needs muscle strength, lean body mass, and reduced body fat, as well as excellent balance and hand-to-eye coordination. I felt that testosterone could be very helpful for her.

It turned out that her most effective dosage caused aggressiveness and acne. The solution was to triple her normal amount of gel on the morning of a surfing competition. Instead of 1 gram of 0.05 percent testosterone gel, she used 3 grams. Then she wouldn't use the gel for up to a week. She experienced no side effects.

This program served Rita well. It is yet another example of how to maximize testosterone-related benefits when you want them. If, like Rita, you have a need for greater power, coordination, and balance, you take the testosterone the day you need it, and take less or none on the days afterward.

A Final Word

Obviously, some people might be tempted to abuse testosterone solely for enhancing physical pleasure. Testosterone is a serious hormone and should be used responsibly under careful medical supervision.

Testosterone is an essential part of my health and antiaging programs. It's the third major addition, after estrogen and progesterone, for building up and strengthening a woman in all aspects of her daily life. The key is finding the right balance. Once you find it, you have a really remarkable tool at your disposal.

Never ignore even the most minimal signs of excess. When they occur, decrease your daily or intermittent dosage until the side effects are gone.

18

Human Growth Hormone

Human Growth Hormone at a Glance

In time, and hopefully soon, human growth hormone (HGH) will fulfill the modern-day search to minimize the ravages of aging. It is definitely one of the "stars" of current antiaging research, as a *New York Times* article said in 1995.

HGH significantly promotes the vitality, maintenance, and integrity of your organs on a systemic basis. Produced by the pituitary gland (the body's master gland), it impacts nearly every cell and stimulates the release of a few hundred growth factors in the body. It also helps other hormones penetrate into the cells and react more efficiently.

Like many other hormones, HGH peaks in the early twenties and then starts on its downward slide. *By the time you reach fifty, you have half the amount you had earlier in life, and if you reach ninety, you have lost 90 percent.*

So fundamental is this hormone to proper physiological functioning, that its decline in the body correlates directly to the aging process. In recognition of this connection, scientists have identified growth hormone deficiency as a specific clinical syndrome.

This table clearly indicates the major impacts of HGH. I regard it as *an essence of youthfulness* involved in everything from organ function to love of life to mental and physical performance.

All you have to do is look at yourself in the mirror and compare what you see now to a photograph of how you looked twenty years ago. At a glance, you see the effect of declining HGH. The wrinkles and creases tell the story, as do the falling cheeks and thinning lips.

Check the elasticity of your skin—another indicator of HGH. Gently pinch the skin on the back of your hand and pull it upward. If it returns slowly, that's a sign of aging skin. With age, the skin becomes thinner and less elastic. On an older person, you can readily separate the skin from the under-lying tissue, something you can't do with children.

Research has primarily focused on physical effects of HGH replacement—

SYMPTOMS AND SIGNS OF GROWTH HORMONE DEFICIENCY IN ADULTS

Symptoms	*Signs*
Impaired psychological well-being and quality of life	Less lean body mass
Poor general health	Less bone mineral density
Less self-control	More body fat
Depression	Decreased HDL cholesterol
Increased anxiety	Increased LDL cholesterol
Less vitality and energy	Lessened kidney function
Impaired emotional reactions	Lowered basal metabolic rate
Increased social isolation	Reduced muscle and strength
Intensified jet lag effect	Reduced exercise/aerobic capacity
Resistant to new ideas and situations	Possibly reduced size of brain
Tendency to habituation	Reduced immune function
	Loss of skin tone

on the bones, skin, fat, and muscle. Most of the studies have failed to *recognize perhaps the most important benefit of HGH: promotion of mental youthfulness. HGH is the fuel of creativity, ability to change and grow, to try, to dare, and to reach new levels. When you lose HGH you lose these qualities. They are replaced with cynicism, negativity, the inability to share, compromise, innovate and expand, and the loss of enthusiasm and inspiration.*

HGH does so much and takes away so much from life when it declines. Yet the name human growth hormone is somewhat misleading. It gives the false impression of making things grow that shouldn't really grow. The real picture is that it promotes growth wherever growth is needed.

Until only recently, HGH as a replacement hormone was only available (and in short supply) by extraction from the pituitary glands of animals and human cadavers. Recombinant DNA technology has changed all that. Today, man has harnessed bacteria to "mass-produce" HGH. Although it is still very expensive, ample HGH is now available for research and therapy.

In laboratory experiments, the hormone has been supplemented to mice and extended their life span by a third.

What does this imply for humans? Stanley Slater, deputy associate director of the National Institute on Aging, told the *New York Times* in 1995 that substances such as human growth hormone that promote growth and maintenance of tissue "may not be the 'fountain of youth' as some have suggested." Yet, he added, "they may have promise for halting or reversing degenerative changes in bones, muscles, nerves and cartilage, which lead to frailty." In his opinion, some type of HGH therapy might help people "stay stronger, leaner and more mobile" in later years.

What the Research Tells Us

Most of the research with HGH involves extremely high doses that had produced exaggerated results along with side effects. As an example, researchers in one recent study gave test subjects thirty-six units of HGH a week. HGH is measured in units. By comparison, most of my patients on HGH receive two to six units a week. Thus, in this study, people received six to eighteen times more than a practical clinical dose.

The researchers concluded that some results were good, but that there were complications, and that growth hormone could possibly induce diabetes. People hear about such studies and they get scared.

Basically, the scientists have taken a natural hormone, used many more times the amount given to patients by clinicians, and then issued a conclusion for caution. For sure, we all need to use any supplement, hormone, or medication with intelligence. This book is not about taking hormones for research purposes, but about replacing your own personal loss of hormones in a safe and balanced way in order to maintain optimum function, promote healthy longevity, and address individual needs.

Benefits of HGH

Used conservatively, HGH generates many exciting and substantial improvements. Here is a short list of them:

- Better muscle tone.
- Improved elasticity of the skin.
- Higher bone density.
- Enhanced immune function.
- More vigor and energy.
- Greater sense of inspiration, zest, creativity, and positivity.
- Mental clarity.
- Reduced irritability.
- A greater sense of friendliness and giving.
- A heightened can-do attitude.
- Less blaming of others.

Availability of HGH

All applications of HGH, including for antiaging purposes, require a prescription. If you are interested in HGH, I recommend seeking out a qualified physician who has been specially trained. The American Academy of Anti-Aging Medicine can provide you with the name of a physician who has completed courses on HGH treatment. The organization is located at 1341 W. Fullerton, Suite 111, Chicago, IL 60614 (Phone: 773–528–4333; on the Internet at www.worldhealth.net).

Research findings have created great enthusiasm and demand for HGH. However, at this point the hormone is relatively expensive. As a result, a growing traffic in HGH sales outside the medical community has developed, along with vigorous marketing of HGH substitutes.

There are many varieties of HGH-type products, ranging from secretagogues, substances that are intended to increase pituitary release of HGH, to homeopathic HGH. They are heavily advertised in bodybuilding and health magazines, as well as on the Internet.

My clinical experience with these HGH substitutes over the last five years is disappointing. Only about 10 percent of my patients who have tried these products have reported benefits and continue to reorder them. I have generally seen little resemblance between the marketing promises and actual results. I should say, however, that I have not checked out every one of them. But I have tested several brands of each type of HGH substitute. Among my colleagues, I have found little enthusiasm for these products as well.

I am not suggesting that these products are bogus. I am only saying that they failed to deliver for the great majority of my patients who have tried them.

I am still waiting for a product that is readily available and affordable for most people. The answer may one day be HGH release factor. This substance, produced by the hypothalamus, stimulates the pituitary secretion of HGH. It's a much simpler molecule than HGH and could be more easily adapted for use as sprays and sublingual drops.

There are two "economy class" methods at the present time to increase your HGH level. The first is through supplementation with certain amino acids that have been individually shown to elevate HGH if taken regularly in high quantities. However, the effect is not as powerful as when taking HGH directly.

The HGH-stimulating amino acids, and their daily doses, are as follows:

- Arginine, 8 grams
- Ornithine, 2.5 grams
- Glutamine, 2 grams
- Lysine, 1.2 grams
- Glycine, 10 grams.

There is no need to take all of them. One will generally suffice. For maximum effect, take the amino acid before sleep and preferably a few hours after eating.

The second inexpensive way to elevate HGH is through exercise, particularly weight training. We all know the importance of regular exercise for good health. Exercise enhances the muscles, bones, and heart. Studies have also shown it can increase your HGH by as much as 20 percent.

Who Should Use HGH

Basically, anyone who can afford it.

Who Should Not Use HGH

People with exhausted adrenal glands should not use HGH. They feel worse after taking HGH. The adrenals produce many hormones, including those that allow your body to respond to stress. When stress is severe and chronic enough, the burden overworks the adrenals and they start to fail. Most doctors don't recognize this condition until it deteriorates into Addison's disease, a serious breakdown in the function of the glands. John F. Kennedy was history's most famous Addison's patient.

Signs of exhausted adrenals include constant daylong fatigue, low blood pressure, faintness when standing up, and feeling "wiped out" after any exertion. Anyone who feels worse with HGH should consult with a physician for an evaluation of adrenal function.

People with cancer should not take HGH. This is primarily a legal medical issue. There is no evidence, either in short-term or long-term studies, showing that low doses of HGH (two to eight units a week) produce an increase in cancer.

Before Starting HGH

Three tests are critical before starting HGH. Your physician who administers HGH is familiar with these testing details. So don't be concerned.

1. **Morning fasting insulin level.** In consideration of the possible effect of HGH on insulin, I have new patients undergo a fasting insulin level test before beginning HGH. If the insulin blood level reads more than 15 mcu/ml, I first put the patient on a supplement and diet program. Refer to the discussion on insulin in chapter 3. Once the insulin level has come down, HGH can be administered.
2. **Morning fasting level of insulin growth factor-1 (IGF-1).** This substance, produced by the liver, is used as the testing indicator for HGH activity. It is one of countless growth factors in the body stimulated by HGH.
3. **The IGFBP3 level, the specific binding protein of IGF-1.**

How Not to Use HGH

As a physician who practices antiaging medicine and who lives in a city where people have a great degree of interest and access to HGH, I see quite a cross section of people using, and often misusing, HGH. I see individuals using very high doses, sometimes as high as twenty times the clinical dose, for the purpose of enhancing muscle development. As a result of this practice, there is real potential to develop thickening of the lips and jaws, as well as carpal tunnel symptoms. This kind of activity is risky, experimental, and should be discouraged.

Some clinicians and researchers look for a certain blood level to determine the appropriate intake of HGH. Initially they described deficiency as anything under 350 ng/ml. More recently, they lowered the level to 300. These numbers are not direct measurements of HGH. They relate to insulin growth factor-1 (IGF-1), one of the more stable substances in the body used to measure HGH activity.

There is a major problem with this approach. The normal range of IGF-1 at age twenty-five is 180 to 780. That's a huge range. More than 50 percent of women before the age of twenty-five will test below 300. Aiming strictly for a blood level minimizes the importance of individuality, which I have spoken about so much in this book.

The Right Way to Use HGH

Thierry Hertoghe, M.D., the Belgian antiaging specialist who has used HGH longer than any other physician for antiaging purposes, has set what I believe to be the most rational standard. He suggests between two to six units per week, a highly effective yet very safe dosage. This dosage model is followed by many antiaging physicians, including myself.

Hertoghe has found that higher doses are unnecessary because HGH has an effect on so many reactions and hormones in the body. Moreover, a conservative dose of HGH, taken in combination with other hormones, achieves results as good as using higher doses of HGH alone.

I have found this to be the case in my practice. In fact, I usually don't recommend HGH alone unless a patient specifically asks for it that way. I much prefer to use it as part of a multifaceted hormone program.

There is yet another reason to stay conservative. There is still a good deal that we don't know about human growth hormone.

HGH is self-administered subcutaneously with the same kind of small needle used by diabetics. Generally, you won't feel any discomfort, even if you are squeamish. The injection zone is a half to one inch on the right or left side of the navel. Pinch the skin gently and insert the needle into the flesh. There are actually a few points in this area where you will hardly feel any sensation at all. An alternative site is the front of the thigh. Inject the hormone just under the skin and not into the muscle tissue.

The physician who supervises your treatment will instruct you on how to administer the HGH. *Be sure to follow a standard sterility technique.*

The best approach, in my opinion, is to mimic nature and administer HGH during its natural peak production time in the body—between 10 to 12 P.M. This is when 90 percent of your HGH is made. There are many smaller pulses throughout the day.

I suggest taking it daily, following the body's own nightly cycle. If you miss a dose, you can double up the next evening. I see no practical reason to take it in divided doses, as some physicians suggest.

Many individuals report a substantial increase in strength, endurance, and energy from taking HGH early in the day. Although this is not a physiologic approach, the daytime response is indeed quick and pronounced.

I personally have taken HGH for some years, usually in the evening before bedtime. On days of travel, extra heavy workloads, or where I have to perform obstetrical duties in the middle of the the night and then go to my clinic in the morning without sleeping, I will often give myself an A.M. injection. I can say from firsthand experience that the effect is quite impressive.

But I leave it to patients to decide the timing that works best for them.

Some physicians recommend doubling the dose and administering HGH every other day. Their fear is that daily administration may suppress your own production. I see no evidence of this in my practice or in the medical literature.

There are a few different preparations of HGH, each with different guidelines.

Regarding the option of using HGH-releasing factor—at the present time it is twice as expensive as HGH. It is also more painful to inject.

The Side Effects

Can you take too much and develop side effects even at conservative doses? Remember, we are all individuals, and indeed the possibility exists.

The first clear sign of excess is water retention, such as experiencing difficulty when putting on or removing a ring. I have never seen this among women taking a dose of two units a week. I have seen it in very few women who use four units, and in about 5 to 10 percent of women on six units a week.

There could be some tingling in the extremities.

Extreme side effects, rare at these doses, include an arthriticlike pain and carpal tunnel syndrome. I have never seen this among patients who use the safe doses I have described.

If you know somebody taking huge doses of HGH, you might want to show them this book. That person may indeed develop bigger muscles and lose body fat. But sooner or later, you will see unsightly thick skin developing and the lips, jaw, and cheeks becoming enlarged. These are features that characterize a rare condition called acromegaly, in which the pituitary gland produces an abnormally high amount of HGH.

In the high-dose medical studies, where researchers used thirty-six units of HGH a week, there was a significant increase in insulin resistance. This means that the cells become less responsive to insulin, which promotes the distribution of glucose to the cells for energy production. This level of HGH is six to eighteen times higher than what I use in my practice. With the low level of usage I recommend you might occasionally see a slight increase in insulin resistance. This can usually be remedied by reducing carbohydrates in the diet.

HGH and Cancer

From time to time patients have asked about growth hormone and cancer. They say they have heard that growth hormone causes cancer.

Again, cancer is not generally a disease of youth. Cancer is usually associated with aging. As the level of HGH declines in the body, the incidence of cancer increases. If HGH promoted cancer, we could expect to see more disease among the young rather than among older people. It seems like common sense to me that a hormone our body utilizes to keep the immune system strong is hardly likely to be the cause of cancer.

I believe that as long as we are cautious and don't overdose with HGH, there is no evidence that replacement can lead to cancer.

The connection between HGH and cancer has been grossly distorted. One misrepresentation relates to acromegaly, the rare condition caused by an overproduction of HGH that I mentioned a moment ago. Individuals with acromegaly have a *slightly* higher incidence of cancer, especially colon cancer.

Another misrepresentation relates to recent studies showing acceleration of cancer growth in *laboratory tests* on isolated animal and human cells. The problem with these studies is that HGH has a positive influence on the whole body, including the immune system. Taking cells out of the body and isolating them from the many systems that HGH affects proves nothing. The clinical fact is that every aspect of immunity improves when you supplement a person with HGH. There are fewer colds and less illness. Chronic conditions and stamina improve.

Other studies have shown rather conclusively that there is no connection between HGH and cancer. Let me cite two of them here:

- Scandinavian researchers monitored HGH-deficient adults for nearly twenty years who had had brain tumors and their pituitary glands removed surgically. One group of patients followed a hormone replacement program that included HGH. The second group followed a replacement program without HGH. There was no difference in cancer recurrence between the two groups.
- HGH was given to a group of youngsters as a growth enhancer. Researchers found no difference in the incidence of leukemia between these young patients and the general population of children.

Monitoring Your Intake with Your Physician

Ideally, you will be working with a knowledgeable physician who can monitor progress and conduct periodic testing every six months.

In most cases there is an increase of 10 to 30 percent in insulin growth factor-1 blood level. I want to make sure at the same time that the specific IGF–binding protein is not elevated. If your HGH treatment were to result in a 20 percent increase of your IGF-1, and at the same time you increase the level of this protein that binds IGF-1 by 20 percent, this is an indication that you haven't really achieved anything.

Keep in mind that you may encounter widely varying test results among different laboratories. There could also be a wide difference in test results from one checkup to the next.

About one-fifth of the individuals using HGH have no significant change in their IGF-1 level. Some researchers suggest this is due to the injected hormone in some way depressing the pituitary gland's own production of HGH. Thus, the thinking goes, there would be less HGH on hand to stimulate IGF-1 release by the liver. I believe the issue is more complex. IGF-1 is just one of a multitude of factors affected by HGH.

If you were to stop the injections in this group of individuals, most of them will report within three months that they no longer feel the positive benefits of HGH. When they resume HGH, they feel the effects again.

There are three things you can do in this situation:

1. Switch to HGH release factor because it stimulates the pituitary to produce more HGH.
2. Administer HGH during the day.
3. Continue with the HGH injections if you feel significant benefits that disappear when the hormone is stopped.

If you are among this group of people and are gaining benefits, I don't see any reason to stop taking the hormone based on a blood test that fluctuates and tracks only one growth factor out of a few hundred. However, this is a personal decision you must make.

What if you take HGH and don't feel a difference? My answer is that this treatment is not only for obvious symptomatic relief. It contributes as well to the health of your bones, liver, kidney, spleen, and lungs. It enhances your immune system. You may or may not witness a magical overnight transformation enveloping your body. With the doses I recommend, the changes are not dramatic, and shouldn't be dramatic. You need to overdose yourself in order to get such drama, and I have explained why that is not in your interest.

Results with HGH

CAROL'S STORY

Here was a forty-two-year-old secretary obsessed with staying thin. She was five-foot-six and 105 pounds. She was not active. She maintained her figure by skipping meals.

Carol was malnourished, with little resistance and energy. She had a protein deficiency. Her cholesterol level was 145 (too low). Remember that cholesterol is the starting point for many of your most important hormones.

She was a good candidate for HGH but was not able to afford it. So we took the alternative route to raise her HGH level.

First, she eliminated most of the carbohydrates in her diet to restore a better insulin picture. She ate only a few low-glycemic index foods a day, concentrating on good sources of protein, fruit, and nuts and seeds (with the exception of peanuts). She stayed away from low-fat foods, which are often loaded with sugar. Twice a week she ate fish.

I had her add four tablespoons of safflower or sunflower oil to obtain omega-6 fatty acids and increase her HDL cholesterol, the "good" cholesterol.

I had her take a combination of 4 grams of arginine, 1 gram of glutamine, and 2 grams of ornithine. These amino acids are know to increase HGH.

She began an exercise program, alternating between running and weight training.

Within six months, Carol was a new person. She had gained only three pounds, which she could live with. But she had become stronger, firmer, more energetic, and more positive and secure about herself and her life. Her skin was more elastic. She looked great.

Her medical tests confirmed the turnaround. Her overall cholesterol went up to a healthier level of 185. Her LDL ("bad") cholesterol dropped, as well as her triglycerides. Her HDL ("good") cholesterol was up. Her fasting level of insulin decreased, meaning her body was handling sugar more efficiently. Her IGF-1 level showed a 35 percent increase, and she was feeling many of the benefits that come from taking HGH.

SARA'S STORY

Sara, forty-four, a vegetarian, came intent on having HGH treatment after reading about the "miracle of human growth hormone." A previous physician had given her HGH, but she felt worse with it. When I did her medical history it became obvious why she had a negative response to HGH.

Sara had fibromyalgia. Pain and fatigue had dominated her life for the previous five years. She had low blood pressure (90 over 60) and always felt dizzy when she stood up. She admitted having difficulty coping with emotional or physical challenges. She reacts in an exaggerated way to every issue she encounters in life, whether large or small, as if the whole universe weighs on her every decision. She described the failure of her son to pass a driving test earlier in the day as if it were an international crisis. Any extra effort exhausts her.

Sara looked older than her years. She had deep wrinkles. Her skin was thinner than normal for her age and had poor elasticity. She had little muscular strength.

All that she told me suggested adrenal exhaustion and a deficiency of HGH. Indeed, her workup showed a very low level of fasting cortisol, a sign of weak adrenals. This was understandable after years of stress from fibromyalgia. She also had high triglycerides and low HDL cholesterol, indicative of hyperinsulinemia.

These findings indicted she was not a candidate for HGH treatment at the present time.

I addressed the adrenal and insulin issues first. Among other things, I decreased her intake of high glycemic index carbohydrates and increased her vegetarian sources of protein, including more soy products.

After three months, we began HGH treatment. I started her on four units a week.

The effect now was extremely positive. Many of her fibromyalgia symptoms improved. She regained long-lost stamina and energy, resistance to colds, and tolerance to stress. Emotionally, she did an about-face, changing from a person who could only do the minimum to someone who now was eager to learn new things. Moreover, every setback was no longer a crisis.

With continued use, there was improvement in skin tone as well.

To be sure, I wasn't giving Sara HGH alone, but the HGH had enhanced the effect of the comprehensive treatment that included adrenal support, testosterone, DHEA, progesterone, and thyroid. HGH can be an all-star and a great team player as well.

ANN'S STORY

Ann, fifty, an actress, was referred to me for HGH treatment by a plastic surgeon. It is well recognized that taking HGH for about two weeks prior to plastic surgery, and for six weeks afterward, significantly improves cosmetic results.

Only in a situation like this do I recommend higher doses, such as eight units a week.

Indeed, in Ann's case, the results of the surgery were magnificent. And, interestingly, she decided to continue taking the hormone. Ann could afford to do so. I reduced her level to four units a week. That was all she needed for a maintenance dose.

"It's a mental and emotional change that I feel the most," she told me. "And I like it. And that's why I want to continue."

Ann said she felt inspired and energized to pursue new challenges in her life, whereas before she was content to sit back and let things come to her.

In her case, as in many others, it is very rewarding to see how this hormone can overhaul entrenched behavioral and emotional patterns. Even as we age chronologically, HGH clearly infuses youthfulness to the mental processes that govern our activities.

MY STORY: UZZI REISS

While this is a book for women, I would like to share my own personal experience with HGH. In short, many of the same benefits my patients report to me are similar to what I feel myself.

First, let me just say that as part of the antiaging program I have developed over twenty years I use all of the hormones described in this book except estrogen. When HGH became available in the mid-1990s, I added it to my personal program.

HGH has added a definite new dimension of mental performance, enthusiasm, and desire to learn that was not there before. At fifty-five, I feel continually inspired to grow in new knowledge.

Many of my friends at the same age are interested in slowing down and even talk of retiring. Yet I feel vital, strong, and more able, it seems, to face the challenges of daily life. My wife says I complain less than before.

Patients who take HGH most often tell me they feel more strength, inspiration, and zest in their lives. I can personally relate to that.

DHEA

DHEA at a Glance

Accompanied by a clamor that often threatened to shatter the sound barrier for marketing hype, DHEA burst out of research anonymity in the mid-1990s to become an overnight superstar in the supplement and anti-aging community.

One major magazine gushed that DHEA "has earned enough respect to break into the national spotlight as the most broadly useful natural medicine in the battle to resist aging." The article envisioned masses of baby boomers reaching their hundreth birthday hale and hearty thanks to this superhormone.

Now, more than five years later, DHEA is still very much an "in" hormone, but the fever has cooled some and we can calmly consider the important and promising role it plays for health and antiaging benefits.

For the record, DHEA is the merciful abbreviation for dehydroepiandrosterone (pronounced dee-hi-dro-epp-ee-ann-dro-stehr-own). It's a hormone manufactured by the adrenal glands, the organ that also makes adrenaline and cortisol.

DHEA's meteoric rise to popularity followed a medical conference in 1995 sponsored by the prestigious New York Academy of Sciences. The conference was entirely dedicated to DHEA research.

At that event, researchers gathered to present and discuss exciting scientific findings on DHEA. Among other things, they had discovered that circulating blood levels of DHEA, and its close sulfate relative DHEAS, decreased progressively and significantly with the passage of time. At age fifty, the adrenals produce half the DHEA they turn out in the midtwenties. Studies showed that we generally lose about 2 percent a year after twenty-five.

DHEAS is the most abundant hormone in the blood. It is simply a DHEA molecule that becomes attached to a sulfate (a combination of sulfur and oxygen) molecule when it is metabolized in the liver.

DHEA is unique to primates—humans, gorillas, and chimpanzees. Animal studies conducted with rodents have shown that supplementation helped prevent obesity, diabetes, cancer and heart disease, stimulate the immune system, and even extend longevity. These observations led investigators to theorize that some of the degenerative changes associated with human aging could be linked to a progressive deficit in circulating DHEA or DHEAS.

Human epidemiological studies further suggested that a higher DHEAS level might benefit longevity and the cardiovascular system. Thus, DHEA and/or DHEAS "may represent biomarkers of healthy aging," wrote John E. Nestler, of the Medical College of Virginia in a special report on the 1995 conference.

DHEA, like so many other hormones, peaks in humans around the age of twenty-five, when we are generally at our lifetime peak of health and vitality. Then it slowly declines. It appears to be involved in regulating the metabolic balances of youth (anabolism). One can readily see the logic of supplementing a major hormone like this. Whether it can truly impact the aging process and help us live longer remains to be seen. There is no consensus for that among researchers.

But recently, a French study reported in the *Proceedings of the National Academy of Sciences* in April 2000, gave an indication of the antiaging benefits. The researchers found that supplementation could reestablish a more youthful level in the body. Among the elderly women in their study they singled out significant improvements in bone turnover, sex drive, and health of the skin.

Problems with the Research

The animal studies with DHEA are quite interesting, but when I look for revelations and guidance from research with humans I become very confused. Most of the studies about "physiological" replacement of declining DHEA have nothing to do with real life. The doses used in these studies range from 25 to 1,600 milligrams over periods from a single day to six months. *For the most part, the doses are far too high and the duration of the studies far too short.*

DHEA is a hormone that is involved at the ground floor of countless biochemical reactions in the body. Its effects are more diffuse than direct, and more cumulative than immediate.

Over the years, I have probably recommended DHEA to more than seven thousand patients. In that time only one of them was able to take more than 100 milligrams without developing major side effects. I managed to give 50 milligrams to only a handful of patients. Only 10 percent could handle more than 25 milligrams. Most tolerate no more than 10 to 15 milligrams. About 10 percent can't even tolerate 5 milligrams.

When I read about the megadoses in the studies I wonder how the researchers accomplish this without causing intolerable side effects. I can assure you that my patients are no different from any other women. They come in all shapes, races, ethnic backgrounds, and ages—a true microcosm of the world. It is thus hard for me to understand and extract any practical information from these human studies. I can't believe that the women who were given these high doses would continue taking them because of the side effects.

The major conclusion I draw from the studies is DHEA is so safe that the researchers are comfortable using it at relatively high doses. When I prescribe DHEA, I rely essentially on my clinical experience and the experience of other physicians who use it routinely.

Signs of DHEA Deficiency

- Stressed.
- Lack of stamina.
- Intolerance to loud noises.
- Constant fatigue.
- Poor mood.
- Decreased immunity.

- Memory loss.
- Lack of pubic hair.
- Poor abdominal muscle support.
- Dry skin and eyes.
- Poor sex drive.

Among patients, it is difficult to link these signs exclusively to DHEA deficiency. DHEA is one of a number of antiaging hormones that drops slowly after we pass our midtwenties. These signs could reflect the dropping level of not just DHEA but of many different hormones.

Signs of DHEA Excess

Some women have a natural excess of DHEA. They tend to have more hair, oilier skin, and a greater incidence of acne. Women who are very hairy by nature should use DHEA very cautiously.

These, and other symptoms, can also develop from taking more DHEA than your body will tolerate. You could become edgy and irritable.

Supplementing with too much DHEA for a prolonged period of time can generate facial hair and loss of head hair. This is a result of some of the DHEA converting to testosterone.

Signs of excess are commonly seen among women with polycystic ovarian syndrome, an inborn hormonal defect that causes overproduction of DHEA and testosterone.

Who Should Take DHEA Supplements

I regard DHEA as a vital cog and major supporting player in a comprehensive antiaging strategy of hormonal replacement therapy.

I routinely recommend it to patients over thirty-five as compensation for the progressive 2 percent-a-year drop in the body's own production. There are certain situations, however, where I suggest it for women even under twenty.

In general, the main objective of supplementation is to try and prevent the physiological deficits believed to be associated with the decline of DHEA in your body. By thirty-five, production is already down by 20 percent from its peak.

Benefits of DHEA

DHEA can be especially beneficial for the following situations:

Stress

This is a cardinal consideration. The more stress you have the more your body consumes DHEA and the less it makes. Often women can tolerate more DHEA than normal when they are under chronic stress.

Low Energy

DHEA contributes to improved energy and stamina.

Anxiety and Depression

DHEA makes you feel better. It acts as an antidepressant and mood elevator.

Poor Immunity

Animal and human studies indicate that DHEA can reinforce the immune system. It significantly improves the antibody response to vaccinations in the elderly. That means more protection.

It also has the potential to reduce lupus symptoms among female patients. A 1994 study by Stanford University researchers on women with mild to moderate systemic lupus erythematosus demonstrated for the first time that DHEA supplementation might be effective in the treatment of an auto-immune disease. Their results included a lessened severity and frequency of rashes, joint pain, headaches, and fatigue. Lupus is a chronic inflammatory illness that can lead to damage of the kidneys, nervous system, joints, and skin.

In this study, the researchers used 200 milligrams daily for up to six months. That's a level of DHEA that my patients do not tolerate. However, I do not treat lupus. Perhaps individuals with this condition can tolerate much higher doses than healthier patients. Whenever I see patients with lupus I encourage them to mention this study to their rheumatologists. Unfortunately, the specialists tend to show little interest in DHEA.

Several studies have associated higher levels of DHEA in the body to a lowered incidence of cancer. One animal study suggested that DHEA could prevent mammary cancer in rats. However, the limited research does not allow us to draw conclusions regarding breast cancer and DHEA.

Some of my patients have told me they heard or read that DHEA actually increases breast cancer. I have never heard of such research. My only comment is that I would not give DHEA alone to a menopausal woman. The reason is that some of the DHEA could convert to estrogen and intensify estrogen dominance.

High Insulin, Hypoglycemia, Diabetes

DHEA may help reverse the metabolic tendency toward diabetes.

The hormone is known to decrease insulin resistance. In doing so, it improves the utilization of blood sugar for energy and helps prevent diabetes.

Cardiovascular

DHEA research in the prevention and treatment of atherosclerosis has yielded both promising and mixed results. In atherosclerosis, deposits of fatty plaque build up on arterial walls, causing a narrowing that can choke off critical flow of nutrients and oxygen to the heart, brain, and elsewhere in the body.

In a 1988 study conducted at Johns Hopkins University, the therapeutic effect of supplemental DHEA was tested on rabbits with severe atherosclerosis. The results: a nearly 50 percent reduction in plaque size among the supplemented animals compared to a control group.

Among humans, epidemiological studies suggest that a higher DHEAS level may mean greater cardioprotection for males, but not for females.

One long-term statistical analysis of 1,029 men and 942 women conducted by researchers at the University of California at San Diego revealed that a higher level of blood DHEAS was associated with a significant 15 to 25 percent reduction in the risk of fatal cardiovascular disease in men. For women, there was a nonsignificant increase in the risk. The analysis involved subjects aged thirty to eighty-eight who were monitored for nearly two decades.

At the New England Research Institutes in Massachusetts, researchers also found that higher levels of DHEA and DHEAS in middle-aged women might indicate an increased cardiovascular risk. Their study was based on 236 women between the ages of fifty to sixty who were monitored from 1986 to 1995.

I believe the findings for women are invalid for a simple reason. About 15 percent of the female population has a condition called polycystic ovarian syndrome. These are women with a naturally high level of DHEA throughout their lives. They also have high levels of cholesterol and insulin. These two factors increase their cardiovascular risk. In my opinion, any study to determine the relationship of DHEA and general female cardiovascular health must exclude these women. Their participation skews the results.

Studies conducted at the Medical College of Virginia indicate that DHEA may retard the platelet aggregation effect in humans and thus offer additional cardiovascular protection. Platelets are structures found in the blood that play a major role in clotting.

Endocrine Function

In one 1994 study, researchers gave women 50 milligrams of DHEA and found that it increased their testosterone and HGH, but not their estrogen level. It decreased the level of SHBG. The practical conclusion is that if you megadose a woman like this you will not increase her estrogen but will increase her testosterone and the availability of HGH to the body.

In one of the most outrageous experiments I have ever seen, researchers gave 1,600 milligrams daily to menopausal women for a month. They found that total cholesterol dropped by 10 percent. The good cholesterol dropped also by 20 percent and there was an increase in the insulin level.

The participants in this study were given a hundred times the usual amount that women can tolerate. I have a hard time envisioning a woman able to tolerate such doses for a month.

In a 1999 study reported in the *New England Journal of Medicine,* German researchers conducted a double-blind study using 50 milligrams of DHEA daily for twenty-four women with adrenal exhaustion. Results from the four-month study showed that the DHEA significantly improved the well-being and sexuality of the participants as well as helped them with anxiety and depression.

Fertility

Researchers gave 80 milligrams of DHEA daily for two months to women under the age of forty-two who did not respond to fertility drugs. They found a 300 percent improvement in their response. In my practice, I suggest that patients with infertility problems try to take as much DHEA as they can tolerate.

Psychological

Researchers believe that the age-related drop in DHEA levels could be involved in behavior, functionality, and mental illnesses. Brain tissue contains five to six times more DHEA than elsewhere in the body.

Evidence points to an apparent relationship between low levels of DHEA and the degeneration of brain cells. This connection is encouraging exploration of DHEA as a potential agent in treating and slowing down senility-associated degenerative disorders, such as Alzheimer's disease.

A 1999 McGill University study examined the DHEA level in twenty-six women with Alzheimer's disease. The researchers determined that a higher level of the hormone corresponded to better mental function.

An earlier study at the University of California at La Jolla found a pronounced improvement in the perception of psychological (and physical) well-being among a small group of elderly men and women taking DHEA supplements for three months.

A strong relationship between low DHEA and depression was found in a study of 699 women aged fifty to ninety living in a Southern California community for seniors. In this 1999 statistical analysis, the researchers concluded that long-term clinical trials of DHEA therapy should be conducted with older women who have depressed moods.

Dry Skin

Studies show that DHEA can improve the moisture level, lubrication, thickness, and pigmentation of the skin.

DHEA Is Not a Prescription Item

DHEA capsules can be purchased from health practitioners, health food stores, drugstores, compounding pharmacies, and through mail order. No prescription is needed.

The hormone is also available as creams/gels or sublingual drops from compounding pharmacies.

Don't be confused by DHEA claims made for steroidlike herbal extracts of wild yams. Promoters of these products describe such products as precursors of DHEA. However, there is no evidence that wild yam supplements raise the blood level of DHEA. Wild yam may have some other benefits as far as a nutritional supplement is concerned, such as tonifying the system, but nothing has been proven yet.

I prefer DHEA supplements prepared by compounding pharmacists or marketed by well-known nutritional supplement companies. That's because I am concerned about the potencies of some products sold over-the-counter or through mail order. One of the leading DHEA researchers decided to analyze some of these products. He discovered many discrepancies between label claims and actual contents. Some products had only 10 percent of the claimed quantity of DHEA.

That's good news and bad news. The good news is that some people are recommending as much as 150 to 200 milligrams for women. This is pure insanity! If there is only 10 percent in the bottle then you may only be getting 15 to 20 milligrams, which is more along the lines of what a woman can tolerate.

But what if the label is accurate? That would be the bad news. Some of my patients can't tolerate more than 1 or 2 milligrams a day.

If you do purchase DHEA over-the-counter, stick to reliable brands and very low doses.

What Kind of DHEA Should You Take?

DHEA can generate different benefits, depending on the form you use.

Oral. Capsules or sublingual drops increase the DHEA and testosterone levels in the blood. The levels reach a peak very fast, stabilize for three months, and afterward drop down by 20 to 25 percent from their peak values.

Most of my patients use either drops or pills. My preference is drops.

Capsules are the easiest form to use, but they tend to increase the testosterone level more frequently compared to sublingual drops.

Capsules create a DHEA peak level in the body in two hours; the sublingual drops in about a half hour.

Topical gels/creams. The disadvantage here is that you have to use about ten to fifteen times more DHEA than you would in the capsule or drop form in order to get the same benefits. Instead of a 10- or 15-milligram capsule, for instance, you would need 100 to 150 milligrams of DHEA in the gel form. That makes it very expensive.

Vaginal creams. This method increases the DHEA level in the body without elevating DHEAS and testosterone. I have no clinical experience using DHEA vaginally.

Before Starting DHEA

I don't recommend DHEA to patients until after doing a blood test for their DHEAS level. DHEAS, you remember, is the more abundant relative of DHEA. It is more stable, has fewer fluctuations, and provides a good marker with which to determine how much DHEA you have.

Among medical laboratories, DHEAS levels are measured in several different concentrations. Typical ranges for a twenty-five-year-old woman at these various concentrations are as follows:

- 65 to 360 ug/dl.
- 0.5 to 4.1 mcg/ml.
- 1,800 to 3,600 mcg/dl.

The initial blood test provides a baseline that can be used when you retest later after starting on DHEA. I recommend checking your blood level again in three months.

Don't start DHEA at the same time you start a thyroid replacement program. Each can cause some edginess if you take an excess. Similarly, don't increase DHEA at the same time you increase your intake of thyroid medication.

How to Take DHEA

DHEAS naturally peaks each day in the body between 6 A.M. and 1 P.M. You should follow this circadian pattern when you supplement with DHEA. Take it in the morning and/or midday.

In many of the high-dose medical studies, DHEA was taken before sleep. *I only recommend this if for some reason you want to stay awake.*

DHEA is fat-soluble. It is better absorbed with a meal, preferably breakfast or lunch, that includes some healthy fat. If you take DHEA at dinnertime you might have trouble falling asleep. If you want to stay awake longer, then take it with dinner.

In general, start at around 5 milligrams daily. Take the DHEA in capsule or drop form. Each drop should equal 1 to 5 milligrams.

If you have a small frame, weigh less than 110 pounds, and have a low blood level of DHEAS (under 60 mcg/dl), I suggest starting with 1-milligram potency drops.

Dosages can be increased every week or two. You can either take more at one time or add a second dose at lunch.

Let's assume that you are fifty years old. Your DHEAS blood level now is 125 mcg/dl, about half the amount you had at twenty-five. Your goal is to try to regain that earlier level.

Such a goal is fine as long as you don't create side effects in the process. Most women will develop oily skin, edginess, or pimples—signs of excess— as soon as they take too much DHEA. If this occurs, stop the DHEA. Wait until the symptoms disappear. Then resume with a lesser amount.

For women who are stressed, depressed, who have diabetes or a high level of insulin, or who are in bodybuilding training, try to take the maximum dose without side effects.

Monitoring Your Intake

Like all hormone replacements, responses to DHEA are very individual. Many women experience all the expected benefits of DHEA. Some quickly, others gradually. Some say they can't attribute any improvements to DHEA. It just depends on how deficient you are to begin with and how your body utilizes it. The issue always comes back to individuality.

From my clinical standpoint, DHEA exerts a pivotal influence in your constitutional makeup. Whether you feel major or minor improvement or nothing at all, the hormone is doing some good at some deep-down level of the physiology.

Among the benefits I listed above, the dominant improvements I see among patients are *mood elevation, mental clarity, gaining energy, stamina, and confidence, and promotion of sexuality.*

DHEA is widely regarded as an aid to promote fat loss and lean body mass, however I have not seen impressive results with my patients. When I work with patients on weight loss, I ask them first to increase their level of healthy dietary fat and decrease carbohydrates. After about two weeks, I recommend starting DHEA. Women on very low fat diets, by the way, have less tolerance for DHEA.

Among my patients are a number of women who, for various reasons, chose only to replace DHEA. Even though they had other deficiencies, they were interested only in DHEA supplementation. I think this is a wrong approach. Yet because DHEA has such a basic role in the body, I knew they would get some benefits.

JEAN'S STORY

One such patient was Jean, forty and infertile. She was relatively fatigued, depressed, and lacking in motivation. She had read about DHEA and wanted me to start her on this hormone alone.

Her baseline DHEAS blood level was about 150. I recommended 5 milligrams to start, taken with breakfast. After two weeks, she was to add another 5 milligrams with lunch. I told her to keep increasing slowly until she took 10 milligrams twice a day.

After six weeks, she reported starting to feel edgy a couple of hours after taking the second dose at lunch. Her limit turned out to be 10 milligrams in the morning and 5 milligrams at lunch.

Her skin became slightly oily, but she felt more enthusiastic, confident, and productive. She had more stamina. Overall, she felt significantly improved. In follow up, her DHEAS level had increased to 225 ug/dl.

MEDITATE—AND ELEVATE—YOUR DHEA

Supplementation is not the only way to raise DHEA levels. In a 1992 study reported in the *Journal of Behavioral Medicine*, DHEAS levels in 326 adult practitioners of Transcendental Meditation (TM) were found to be significantly higher than a control group matched for age and sex. The differences were the largest for the oldest age categories.

Stress decreases the body's production of DHEA while at the same time increasing the consumption. Meditation is a powerful tool for stress reduction. Thus, by reducing stress it helps to keep the stress hormone cortisol low and the DHEA high.

20

Melatonin

WHAT'S IN THIS CHAPTER

- Melatonin at a glance
- Benefits of melatonin
- Melatonin is not a prescription item
- Who should take melatonin
- Who should not take melatonin
- Side effects from excess melatonin
- How to take melatonin
- Monitoring your intake

Melatonin at a Glance

It's been called the "superhormone," has appeared on the front cover of *Newsweek* magazine, and been the subject of a best-selling book. According to some companies that market it, it is supposed to help you grow younger at any age, add a decade to your life, and maintain vigor to one hundred years of age.

Behind such exaggerated claims is a very important natural substance that deserves serious consideration as a supplement to any health and antiaging program.

Melatonin is secreted by the pineal, a light-sensitive gland embedded deep in the brain that controls the body's biological clock. It acts as the synchronizer of the whole hormonal-immune network, according to Italian researcher Walter Pierpaoli, M.D., an internationally renowned pineal expert.

Melatonin follows a natural sleep/wake cycle called the circadian rhythm. In this pattern, the level of the hormone rises in your body with darkness and falls with light. The natural peak level is around midnight. A young and healthy pineal turns out 2.5 milligrams of the hormone every twenty-four hours.

Melatonin plays a central role in the natural aging process of the body. Around the age of forty, the pineal production starts to diminish. This decline sets in motion a shift in the way the cells of the body operate. The physiology now moves from a primary mode of repair and rejuvenation to one of aging and degeneration. From this you can readily understand the potential of melatonin replacement.

Pineal expert Pierpaoli believes that degenerative and aging-related diseases, including arteriosclerosis, autoimmunity, immunodepression, cancer, and metabolic conditions, are promoted by a de-synchronization of the hormonal system. By de-synchronization he means loss of cyclicity. And this, he says, is caused by the accelerated or programmed decay of the pineal.

The aging connection was dramatically demonstrated in classical experiments conducted by Pierpaoli. The research was described in the 1995 bestselling book *The Melatonin Miracle* (Pocket Books), written with William Regelson, M.D., of Virginia Commonwealth University.

By adding melatonin to the drinking water of laboratory animals, life span was extended by 30 percent. Older mice became more vigorous and healthier on the "spiked" water.

Pierpaoli also transplanted pineal glands from younger mice into older mice. The older rodents lived much longer than expected. Young mice who received glands from older mice died much earlier than expected.

While there have been no long-term studies on whether melatonin can extend human life, the prospect fascinates consumers and researchers alike.

Today, Pierpaoli is not as sure that the aging benefits he saw in the animal experiments are due entirely to melatonin. He feels there may possibly be other "not yet identified agents" in the pineal that are also involved.

At a recent medical conference, Pierpaoli revealed some rather fascinating facts about the influence of light on pineal production of melatonin. Darkness, as we know, triggers the circadian surge of melatonin in the body. But if you wake up at night and switch on the light in your bedroom, you are also basically switching off your pineal gland.

Pierpaoli also suggested that the brightly lit homes and offices in the United States, compared to a lower lighting standard in Europe, could create a negative effect on health. Our bodies never evolved on so much artificial light, he pointed out.

In northern countries, where winter days have much longer hours of darkness, the production of melatonin is stretched out. This reduces its sleep-time benefits to the body. Seasonal affective disorder (SAD), a condition characterized by depression during winter months, is thought to be related.

Researchers have found that the natural level of melatonin is lower in people with asthma. The sleeping pill decreases production, as do medications such as Clonidine and beta-blockers.

Benefits of Melatonin

Melatonin offers many important and practical benefits.

Sleep. The most celebrated use of melatonin is for sleep. In a 1995 cover article on melatonin, *Newsweek* magazine referred to it as "the all-natural nightcap."

As we get older, our sleep cycle changes significantly. We don't fall asleep as easily. We wake up more frequently. We don't sleep as deeply. And we don't dream as much. These are signs of aging.

Here's how melatonin can help:

1. It decreases the cortisol level in the body. Remember that cortisol is produced by the adrenal glands in response to stress. High cortisol destroys brain cells, accelerates aging, and contributes to sleeplessness.
2. It promotes deep sleep, a significant antiaging benefit.

Jet lag. In the 1980s, research by Josephine Arendt, of the University of Surrey in England, first brought attention to the use of melatonin for relieving jet lag. Subsequent research confirmed the benefit. Reports in the *Wall Street Journal, Business Week,* and many other popular publications soon made melatonin a big hit with airline crews and travelers the world over.

Antioxidant strength. Medical studies show that melatonin may be one of the strongest antioxidants in the body, meaning that it combats the damaging effects of free radicals. In particular, melatonin neutralizes the hydroxyl radical, one of the most harmful types.

Melatonin offers preventive and therapeutic support against cancer. Many studies report significant benefits in breast and prostate cancer with high doses of melatonin, ten to fifty times higher than commonly used doses. The data are very impressive.

The studies also include results showing melatonin can enhance the effectiveness of chemotherapy and reduce its toxicity.

- **Protection of DNA.**
- **Decreases anxiety.** Melatonin stimulates GABA, the brain chemical that calms and relaxes.
- **Bone protection.**
- **Reduction of blood coagulation.**
- **Increases natural killer cell activity.** These cells are among the most important immune factors.
- **Enhances production of T3, the most important thyroid hormone.**
- **Promotes zinc utilization.**
- **Maintains hair color—slows down graying.**

Melatonin Is Not a Prescription Item

Modern chemistry has synthesized melatonin. The supplement you buy in health food stores and drugstores is identical in structure to your own melatonin.

It is available as capsules, sublingual drops, and pills, and as an oral spray. All of these forms are fine.

Who Should Take Melatonin

The multifaceted benefits of melatonin should encourage anyone over the age of forty to take this hormone. It can also be used for specific purposes spelled out in this chapter.

Who Should Not Take Melatonin

Individuals with exhausted adrenal glands should not take melatonin. Such people tend to be constantly fatigued, have low blood pressure, and feel faint when they stand up. They have low tolerance for physical and emotional stress. Melatonin can reduce the production of cortisol and is contraindicated here. Anyone who experiences reduced energy and stamina after taking melatonin should suspect the presence of exhausted adrenals and have their adrenal function evaluated by a physician. Melatonin should not be taken until the adrenals are healthy again.

Women trying to conceive should not take melatonin. It could negatively affect the ovulation process. Melatonin is naturally lower during ovulation.

Side Effects from Excess Melatonin

If you take too much melatonin, you may experience the following effects.

- Drowsiness upon arising.
- Wild dreams. I don't mean vivid dreams. If a patient says she dreams her husband is running after her with a bouquet of roses, that is a pleasant, vivid dream. If she says a gorilla is chasing her with a club, that's a sign of too much melatonin.
- An excess of the thyroid hormone (T3), resulting in waking up nervous, sweating, and with palpitations.
- Decreased estrogen and progesterone levels. One Dutch study suggested that 30 milligrams of melatonin daily could even act as a contraceptive. This effect has not been tested in a large study, however.

How to Take Melatonin

For Sleep

For most people, melatonin acts as a natural, nonaddictive sleeping pill. Regular users range from insomniacs who want to avoid taking sedatives to individuals who simply want a deeper sleep.

In the varied sublingual and oral spray forms, take melatonin ten to thirty minutes before bedtime; for oral capsules, thirty to sixty minutes before.

Start with 1 milligram. Increase by 1-milligram increments daily as needed to reach your desired sleep effect, or until you develop side effects.

Melatonin alone may not always achieve your sleep goals. You may need to utilize other hormones, as I have described elsewhere in the book. Estrogen and progesterone, in balance, have a major benefit for sleep among menopausal women.

Ideally, the room you sleep in should be dark.

Jet Lag

According to Pierpaoli and Regelson, taking 3 to 5 milligrams prior to bedtime after arrival in the new time zone may help minimize jet lag symptoms. If one awakens in the middle of the night, another 3 to 5 milligrams can be taken to promote drowsiness. This approach can be used for several days to assist in resetting the biological clock. On your return home take the same amount before your normal bedtime to help your body readjust.

"Most people find that by following this simple regimen they no longer experience the symptoms normally associated with crossing time zones," Pierpaoli and Regelson say.

Melatonin is often used incorrectly and as a result doesn't provide relief against jet lag. By incorrectly, I mean using it in an environment of bright light. If you take it, for instance, in an airplane that is brightly lit, it won't work as well. Cover your eyes first so that no light comes through. A half hour later, take melatonin. This puts your body in a "melatonin mode" and promotes the effect of the supplement.

For Antiaging

Start with 0.25 to 0.5 milligrams and increase gradually until you develop a side effect. Take melatonin before sleep. An optimum dose is usually 1 to 5 milligrams.

For Cancer Protection

Take 20 to 40 milligrams daily. It is interesting to note that participants in studies using these very high doses did not develop the side effects I described previously. The side effects are associated with much lower doses. Apparently the cellular receptor sites for melatonin become flooded after a certain level.

Monitoring Your Intake

I don't believe monitoring is necessary other than watching for side effects and following your own intuition. Saliva tests are available through your physician if you want to determine a deficiency.

21

Pregnenolone

Pregnenolone at a Glance

Pregnenolone, a hormone produced by the adrenal glands, is regarded as the *mother of hormones*. This claim to fame comes from the fact that when the body creates hormones from cholesterol, the first off the assembly line, so to speak, is pregnenolone. The body further metabolizes pregnenolone into progesterone and DHEA, which then contribute to a widening sequence of hormonal transformations (see the chart on the sequence of hormonal production in chapter 1).

Pregnenolone was first explored during the 1940s as a therapeutic agent in the treatment of a number of conditions, including rheumatoid arthritis. But medical attention soon turned elsewhere with the exciting discovery of cortisone, which delivered quick relief from arthritis and pain.

It wasn't until the 1990s that the name of pregnenolone surfaced again, largely in connection with the popularity of DHEA. However, research lags behind other hormones.

The secretion of pregnenolone falls with age. At fifty, we generally have half the amount of the hormone that we had at twenty-five.

Pregnenolone doesn't really generate a specific set of deficiency symptoms. It operates at a more subtle and supportive level in the physiology. I call it a *silent partner*. After using it for some eight years in my practice, I can't really look at a patient and tell if she is deficient in pregnenolone.

There are very few instances when the addition of pregnenolone makes a significant and dramatic change in someone's condition. Theoretically, when a person takes supplemental pregnenolone it should enhance the conversion process to other hormones and contribute to a restoration of deficient hormones. But I haven't seen any direct evidence of this to date, either in younger or older women. Still, pregnenolone appears to have a subtle and positive effect on all the hormones in the body without creating overtly dramatic improvements.

Clinical experience so far with this hormone among antiaging physicians suggests that we are only beginning to learn how to make potentially significant use of it. We are just getting glimpses of its ability to improve health on a number of different fronts. Pregnenolone appears to have very promising applications for stress, connective tissue, and degenerative disorders. Specifically, it may offer major benefits against chronic fatigue syndrome, arthritis, lupus, ulcerative colitis, and inflammatory bowel disorders.

Pregnenolone Is Not a Prescription Item

Pregnenolone is available as an over-the-counter supplement at health food stores and many drugstores, as well as through compounding pharmacies.

I recommend to patients that they purchase their pregnenolone through a compounding pharmacy where the quality and potency of the product can be trusted.

Many decide, however, to buy an over-the-counter product for the sake of convenience. But buyer beware! OTC products may not have the potency described on the label. If you purchase pregnenolone in this manner, my advice is to stick to well-known brands.

Benefits of Pregnenolone Supplementation

Research shows that pregnenolone supplementation benefits three major areas: the brain, adrenal health, and immunity.

Brain

The data indicates that the hormone can contribute to increased intelligence, learning ability, alertness, memory, and the feeling of well-being. It may help reduce the emotional symptoms of PMS.

A study conducted by the National Institutes of Mental Health found that individuals with depression had a lower-than-normal level of pregnenolone in the fluid that bathes the brain.

In *The Superhormone Promise* (Pocket Books, 1997), William Regelson, M.D., suggests restoration of hormones such as pregnenolone to their youthful levels. This may help prevent "many of the cases of depression that occur among older people and that are all too frequently written off as part of the 'normal' aging process," he says.

Pregnenolone also helps improve vision, and particularly the ability to discriminate among colors.

Adrenal Health

Pregnenolone is considered an antistress hormone. Stress causes the body to produce less and utilize more pregnenolone.

For individuals who lead stressful lives, pregnenolone protects the adrenal glands and helps to maintain balance.

Immunity

Years ago pregnenolone was found to help against rheumatoid arthritis, an autoimmune condition. Patients reported less pain and fatigue and more strength. The effects are not immediate but are felt after some weeks, according to reports from more than fifty years ago.

Who Should Take Pregnenolone

I regard pregnenolone as an unheralded team player that potentiates other hormones. I recommend it to anyone starting a total hormonal replacement program or who has memory or stamina problems.

My main reason for using this hormone is that it occupies such a central position in the hormonal hierarchy.

Many times I find that pregnenolone enhances the benefits of DHEA (see chapter 19) among patients who are unable to take the needed level of DHEA to be effective. Let's say that a woman uses DHEA to improve her stamina. She reaches a certain level but still desires more stamina. If she were to increase her intake of DHEA she would develop side effects. She might get edgy, break out, and her skin become oily. Adding pregnenolone enables her to optimize the effect of DHEA and reach her goal without side effects.

I also recommend pregnenolone for women who want to improve their mental alertness and memory. This hormone is a good place to start the process of memory enhancement.

It also works to support any program for depression or severe PMS that hasn't been totally resolved. Many times, pregnenolone can generate the final extra degree of improvement.

How to Take Pregnenolone

Pregnenolone is available as 50-milligram capsules at health food and drugstores. You can purchase capsules, as well as sublingual drops (5 to 10 milligrams per drop), through compounding pharmacies.

I recommend 50 to 100 milligrams once a day at breakfast. Absorption is better if the meal has some fat in it.

In my practice I also incorporate pregnenolone in a moisturizing cream formula.

Monitoring Your Intake with Your Physician

It is probably a good idea to obtain a baseline blood level before starting pregnenolone.

After three months I suggest another blood level test based on a blood draw six hours after you take the hormone. Normal blood levels are 70 to 120 ng/dl.

If you take too much, you may feel some edginess. That is the only side effect that I have seen at dosages up to 250 milligrams daily. Pregnenolone can be increased gradually in 50-milligram increments. If you see no improvement or you develop any discomfort, return to a lower dosage.

PART FIVE

Putting It All Together

22

How to Take Multiple Hormones

DENISE'S STORY

Denise, forty-three, was a very dynamic businesswoman, the successful owner of a chic clothing boutique in Beverly Hills. She was married with two children. But her world was coming apart.

"My problems started twelve years ago after the birth of my second child," she related. "I developed severe postpartum depression, lost quite a bit of hair, and never could shed a lot of the weight that I gained during the pregnancy."

Denise then proceeded to detail a cascade of increasing health and emotional problems.

Nine months after her last child was born and at the end of her maternity leave, she started developing PMS problems that eventually became more severe. She had anxiety, mood swings, water retention, and an insatiable craving for chocolate. She started having friction with her husband and employees, and being impatient with her children.

217

Her physician recommended antidepressants and antianxiety pills. They helped take some of the edge off but seemed also to make her more fatigued.

She felt she needed a regimented exercise program to restore lost zest, energy, and muscle tone, as well as to help her lose more weight. She was still carrying fifteen pounds more than her prepregnancy weight. At age thirty-five, she started working with a personal trainer. She made some progress but much less than her expectations.

Denise's depression and anxiety worsened. Her interest in sex was decreasing. Her marital discord was growing. She was finding that the stresses of child rearing and work were becoming overwhelming. She was taking more and more time off from work, leaving a manager increasingly in charge, and finding herself less motivated to explore new and exciting lines for her boutique.

"I went from being a strong, take-charge person adept at handling the daily stresses of life to somebody suddenly overwhelmed by everything," she told me. "I became very insecure. My responses to people and situations were often improper. I required constant reinforcement. I was pretty miserable and I'm afraid I made others around me miserable as well. I didn't like what I had become."

In the six months before she came to see me, Denise said that she had to stop working. She had deeper episodes of depression. She found it difficult to fall asleep. She lacked motivation particularly before and during her period. She was taking Prozac, sleeping pills, and tranquilizers.

"The only time I seem to be able to relate well to my universe is the second week into my cycle," she said.

Denise's story strongly suggested a domino effect of hormonal imbalance.

The postpartum depression, hair loss, and inability to shed much of the weight gain from her last pregnancy appeared to be a typical postpartum deficiency in progesterone and thyroid. This combination of deficiencies could have set the stage for the PMS symptoms that started when her period resumed after childbirth.

Her attempts to build up stamina and lose weight had failed possibly because of lack of DHEA, testosterone, and thyroid hormone. She had increasing stress. This probably caused a drain on her DHEA, which is a critical hormone for adrenal health. The adrenals produce the body's stress hormones.

Her description of new symptoms during the last six months sounded like she had now developed signs of estrogen deficiency. These included difficulty in falling asleep, deeper depression, and a growing feeling of doom.

"What you are telling me is understandable from a hormonal perspective," I tried to reassure her. "There are a lot of pieces in your hormonal puzzle and with time I think we can put them in place and restore your balance and whole-ness."

A hormonal workup showed the following:

- Her adrenal function was normal.
- She had no metabolic tendency toward diabetes. Her insulin level was 7 mcu/ml.
- She was thyroid deficient.
- She was deficient in progesterone. On day twenty-five of her cycle, her level was only 6 ng/ml.
- DHEA was low (50 mcg/dl).
- Pregnenolone was relatively low (under 20 ng/dl).
- She was relatively low in human growth hormone, with an IGH-1 level of 125 ng/ml.
- Her estrogen (E2) level showed a major fluctuation, from 250 pg/ml on day twenty of the cycle, down to 24 pg/ml on the second day of the cycle. Her FSH was normal.

In this particular case, my clinical suspicions were confirmed by the lab tests.

My treatment plan called for a multiple hormone approach. First I wanted to restore thyroid balance to her body. I recommended 30 milligrams ($^1/_2$ grain) daily of Armour Thyroid to be chewed upon arising in the morning and before any food is eaten. I asked her to slowly increase the dose until she took a max-imum of 90 milligrams ($1^1/_2$ grains). If she developed any sign of excess, such as palpitations, tremors, edginess, or profuse sweating, I told her to cut back and see me again for a reevaluation.

When she returned to the office in a month, she was quite optimistic.

"My nails are growing. I'm losing less hair. I actually lost two pounds. I have a little more energy. My mood is a little better," she reported.

"This is good news," I said. "Now, let's move forward to the next step. I would like you to start taking estrogen and progesterone sublingual drops."

I recommended Tri-Est estrogen replacement (0.625 milligrams per drop) from day twenty-one to day seven (covering the last and first weeks of the cycle). I wanted her to take one to four drops of estrogen twice a day, increas-ing the amount before her period, and then decreasing after the fourth day of her period. I prescribed eight to twelve drops of progesterone at night and four to six drops at breakfast or lunch. I advised her how to increase or decrease the dosages depending on her symptoms of PMS.

She was to take progesterone from day fifteen to day twenty-eight.

Two weeks later she called to tell me she was feeling much better, except for a slight "spinning" sensation in the morning. I suggested she cut back a bit on her morning dose of progesterone. An excess of progesterone may produce some drowsiness or a spinning sensation.

When she returned to the office for another follow-up in six weeks, she was clearly a transformed woman.

"For the first time in years I am beginning to feel that I have my body, my mind, and my spirit back in sync," she said. "There were times I felt I was going mad, or I would sink to such depths of depression."

Still, she admitted feeling somewhat insecure and lacking the confidence, physical strength, and stamina she was used to in previous years.

"We have managed to achieve a good deal of restoration of your health," I told her. "It's up to you now if you want to go further on a hormonal program. If you do, I would suggest pregnenolone and testosterone."

Pregnenolone would help her overall hormonal stability, while testosterone would be more specific for building up her physical strength, stamina, and confidence. I told her it would also improve her sex drive, which she admitted was still lacking. The relationship between her and her husband was still somewhat shaky after years of friction.

Several months later, Denise said she felt strong enough now to get back full-time into all her usual activities. She wanted to know what the hormonal war chest offered to give her a further boost. I suggested DHEA to help her deal with the stress involved in expanding her activities. I also recommended human growth hormone to support her renewed enthusiasm.

Several months later, Denise returned for an office visit.

"I really feel like a new woman," she reported. "Things are better with my husband and me. And I am back to my old dynamic self. I am playing tennis. I am enjoying my business life and my personal life. I like how I feel and how I look."

Indeed, the person sitting in front of me now was a new woman. She was trim and energetic and radiated health and positivity.

"I still need a bit of medication once in a while to keep the anxiety level down, but I know I will be able to eliminate that someday soon," she said.

A year later, Denise continues to do very well on a program of multiple hormones. She is an obvious success story. She learned to balance and optimize her hormones and turn her life around.

Not every woman has the same ability.

But many do.

And not every case results in such clear-cut improvement.
But many do.

Why Take Multiple Hormones?

The answer is very simple. We are not one-hormone creatures. *We were given a multitude of hormones to carry out a multitude of functions in our body.* Why shouldn't we try to balance and optimize the major hormones in our body as we learn more about their connection to health and aging?

You don't necessarily have to replace all hormones described in this book. The number of hormones my patients take depends on their constitution, symptoms, and goals.

Some women can easily handle multiple hormones, others cannot.

Some are interested in only one hormone for a specific effect.

Others want only to balance estrogen and progesterone.

Others seek a wider spectrum of antiaging benefits from additional hormones.

No matter how many hormones you decide to use, patience and staying in tune with your body's responses are the keys to success.

Belgian physician Thierry Hertoghe, M.D., a fourth-generation endocrinologist and the leading antiaging hormone specialist in the world, believes that the more hormones you use in a replacement program the less quantity you need of each. The reason for this is that they have synergistic and overlapping effects in the body. By improving the system with one, you need less of another to make further improvements. And when you use less of each hormone, the chances of side effects are reduced.

After twenty years in medical practice, this is definitely my clinical observation as well. I have no doubt that the more hormones a patient uses, the better she feels and looks.

Before You Start Taking Multiple Hormones

There are several important steps I strongly recommend before starting a hormonal program. These steps will maximize results, whether you take one or more hormones.

- The first is to maintain healthy levels of cortisol, the stress hormone, and insulin, the pancreatic hormone that governs blood sugar. Refer to chapter 3 for my commentary on these hormones.

- The second step is to be sure that your thyroid is functioning optimally. If you have one or more of the classic signs of thyroid deficiency, you *are* indeed deficient to some degree, even if a blood test shows your thyroid level within a normal range. Common signs of deficiency are as follows: constant feeling of coldness, cold extremities, chronic fatigue, inability to sweat readily from physical exertion, thinning hair, brittle nails, difficulty losing weight, sluggishness in the morning, constipation, dry skin, and a tendency to depression that doesn't respond to medication. Your physician can test you for a deficiency and provide a standard thyroid prescription if you are deficient. To learn more about the thyroid, I recommend Dr. Sanford Siegal's *Is Your Thyroid Making You Fat?* (Warner Books).

- The third step is to follow a diet that supports the hormonal changes you are seeking. Hormones are modulated in the body by fats. If a person eliminates fats from the diet, or eats only one type of fat, the body cannot readily process the new hormonal input. Some of the hormones described in this book should be taken with meals that include healthy fats. Women need to eat a variety of good omega-3, -6, and -9 fats, obtained from sources such as safflower and sunflower oil, butter, eggs, fish, dairy, avocados, nuts and seeds, and certain meats. Fried foods, hydrogenated fats, canola oil, and peanut oil are not in the interest of good hormonal health and longevity.

- Obviously, prior to starting any hormonal program, have a complete physical evaluation by your family doctor and gynecologist.

General Tips

- With the exception of estrogen and progesterone, add other hormones *six to eight weeks apart*. By doing so, you give yourself adequate time to balance each hormone before you add another.

- *At first, use each hormone supplement individually.* Once you are comfortable using more than one at a time, you may want to combine them in a single capsule, gel, or sublingual drop form. Your compounding pharmacist can advise you on combination products.

- When you combine multiple hormones in capsules, creams, and drops, the individual impact of each hormone is somewhat reduced. However, as I mentioned above, there is a synergistic benefit.

- *The same hormone prepared by different compounding pharmacies could generate a different response in your body.* This is because pharmacists use a variety of agents in the product to help "deliver" the hormone into the body. For instance, different oils may be used to enhance the absorption of fat-

SEQUENCE OF TAKING HORMONES

Be sure to familiarize yourself with the details on how to adjust each particular hormone. Remember that you are not a robot. Listen to your body. Adjust accordingly. Don't feel frustrated when you need to change a dosage. Be patient.

1. Estrogen and Progesterone

These are the essential female hormones. *Restoring balance is a priority if deficiencies exist, or if you experience symptoms due to major fluctuations.*

Refer to part two on estrogen, and part three on taking progesterone alone or in conjunction with estrogen.

2. Identify and Address Your Core Concerns with the Appropriate Hormone

You can utilize different hormones to address different problems. Replace the hormones first that relate to your primary concerns.

Refer to the benefits of specific hormones in the section below on deficiencies and symptoms.

3. Total or Multiple Hormone Replacement If You Have No Symptoms

- **Estrogen and progesterone.**
- **Testosterone and human growth hormone.** These two hormones complement each other. They have *totally different* and easily recognizable side effects. Their activities are synergistic.
- **DHEA and pregnenolone.** These adrenal hormones are also synergistic. For someone who has any degree of adrenal insufficiency, DHEA and pregnenolone will be very beneficial. *DHEA should never be started at the same time as testosterone* because the two hormones can produce similar side effects.

soluble hormones. *I have found the differences particularly noticeable with estrogen gels and creams.*

Regarding OTC hormones, actual potencies might vary from what is written on the label. Be aware that you may not be getting what you think you are getting. Stick to well-known brand names.

- If you decide to switch from capsules to sublingual drops or to a gel/cream form of a particular hormone, *you often have to go through a period of readjustment.* That's because each form has a different rate of absorption.

- *Your body may need different doses of different hormones at different times.* When you undergo a prolonged period of stress, for example, you may need more of an individual hormone than at other times.
- *Always remember the individuality factor.* I can't emphasize it enough. The same dose that works perfectly well for your sister or friend may be too much or too little for you.

Specific Hormones for Specific Symptoms and Signs

Poor Physical Appearance and Skin Tone
- Estrogen.
- Human growth hormone.
- Testosterone.
- A special facial hormonal cream can also be obtained from your compounding pharmacist. The one I recommend to patients contains estriol, progesterone, pregnenolone, plus antioxidants.

Prematurely Aged Appearance
- All hormones.

Poor Muscular Definition
- Testosterone.
- DHEA.
- Human growth hormone.

Lack of Energy
- Optimize your thyroid.
- Estrogen, if signs of deficiency exist.
- Provide adrenal support with DHEA and pregnenolone.
- Human growth hormone.

Excess Weight
- Optimize thyroid. If deficient in thyroid hormone (T3), take melatonin.
- Avoid high sex hormone–binding globulin by changing from estrogen capsules or drops to gel.
- DHEA.
- Testosterone.
- Human growth hormone.

Difficulty Sleeping
- Estrogen, if signs of deficiency exist.
- Progesterone.
- Melatonin.
- Human growth hormone.

Poor Sex Drive
- Testosterone, systemically and locally.
- Dihydrotestosterone (DHT).
- DHEA.
- Estrogen, if there are signs of deficiency.
- Medical research suggests that supplementation with human growth hormone and melatonin can increase performance if these hormones are deficient. These hormones have not helped many of my patients for this purpose.

Poor Vaginal Lubrication
- Estriol (E3) vaginally and, if needed, a systemic form of estrogen. About a quarter of my estrogen replacement patients who take capsules or sublingual drops also need to add estriol vaginally for a good lubrication effect.

Memory Loss
- Estrogen, if there are signs of deficiency.
- Pregnenolone.
- DHEA.
- Melatonin.
- Human growth hormone.

Depression
- Always think estrogen first, and particularly if there are signs of deficiency. Young women who are tall, thin, and small-breasted should always give estrogen a chance. For women over thirty-five, a trial of estrogen is always worthwhile, even if the blood level appears to be "normal." By this age there has already been a reduction in the amount of estrogen the body produces compared to earlier years.
- DHEA.
- Pregnenolone.
- Human growth hormone.

Anxiety

- Progesterone. If you are already using progesterone and still have anxiety, try to increase the dosage without incurring side effects.
- Human growth hormone.
- Avoid excesses of estrogen, testosterone, and DHEA. An excess of any of these can increase anxiety.

Migraines

- If they develop before your period, use estrogen and progesterone. If they develop during your period, take estrogen.

PMS

- Progesterone.
- Estrogen.
- Pregnenolone.
- Thyroid, if have signs of deficiency.

Weak Immunity

- Human growth hormone.
- DHEA.
- Melatonin.
- Progesterone.

Osteoporosis

- Progesterone and testosterone. Without any doubt, both of these hormones are more important than estrogen. Estrogen slows down the loss of old bone tissue, but it also slows down the development of new bone. Progesterone and testosterone promote new bone growth and removal of old bone cells.
- Human growth hormone and melatonin are also beneficial.

Using Hormones for "Special Effects"

Over the years, many of my patients have become extremely skilled at achieving "special effects" with natural hormones. By that I mean stepping up their doses to create immediate physical, mental, or mood modifications to meet specific challenges in their lives. The feedback from patients clearly demonstrates that natural hormones can serve as great tools for personal empowerment.

Hormones should only be applied in this way once you have a solid familiarity with them and know how each one affects you individually. Refer to the respective chapter on each hormone. Read the information on signs of excess and how to monitor the hormone.

Testosterone for Strength, Security, Assertiveness, Hand-to-Eye Coordination

To prevent side effects take two to three times the regular daily dose for a day or two. Then stop for a week or ten days.

Here is what some of my patients have reported about the benefits of testosterone:

Rita, a surfer—"Before a competition, I triple my testosterone. By doing that I seem to have triple the balance."

Suzanne, a lawyer—"I double my dosage of testosterone on court days. I feel stronger and more assertive, and have more staying power to get me through exhausting days."

Brenda, a writer—"I see my out-of-town boyfriend every other weekend. On the weekends that we meet I triple up on my testosterone, and then stop for five days."

Deborah, a fitness enthusiast—"I lift weights three times a week. On those days, I double my dose of testosterone a half hour before exercise for added strength."

DHEA and Pregnenolone for Stress Resistance, Endurance, Stamina, and Resiliency

Take them together. They are more likely to generate subtle, rather than immediate effects, although many of my patients increase them before any situation that requires endurance, stamina, and resiliency. Typical uses include prolonged exercise and physical exertion, emotional stress, a long trip, and overcoming colds and flu.

Kim, a college student—"I double my dosage the day before an exam. I find that I can concentrate better. I also take a double amount the day of the exam."

In times of stress, your body may be able to tolerate more of both hormones. But don't increase the amount for longer than a few days at any one time. Afterward, return to your regular dosage. Even a small increase of DHEA can create some edginess.

Human Growth Hormone for Endurance and Enhanced Resistance

If you face a long trip where you cross multiple time zones, or face pro-longed emotional or physical stress, double your daily dose for one or two days.

Please experiment first with the higher doses before you actually use it for a specific situation. While scaling the summit of a mountain peak you don't want to start developing water retention or arthriticlike pains. Some people who take high doses can experience such side effects within forty-eight hours.

HGH can enhance the results of plastic surgery. Take six or eight units a week for two weeks prior to the procedure, and for six weeks afterward.

Progesterone for Calmness and Relaxation

Progesterone stimulates GABA, the major inhibitory neurotransmitter in the nervous system, giving rise to an increased feeling of relaxation. Many of my patients have learned how to adjust the dosage in order to achieve calm-ness throughout the day or whenever needed. But again, please experiment with the hormone first so as not to induce drowsiness when your intention is calmness.

Melatonin for Sleep and Jet Lag

See chapter 20 on how to effectively use this remarkable hormone.

23

Breast Cancer and Hormones

Breast cancer is an extremely emotional and complicated issue. Unfortunately, the relationship between cancer and hormones has been tragically misreported to women. As we continually look for causes, estrogen has become the new scapegoat. If you listen to the media and some of the so-called medical experts, you begin to believe that hormones are carcinogens and that estrogen is on trial. You have to hear patients as I do every day to understand the degree of confusion and fear that exists among women.

Your hormones, I can assure you, are not agents of self-destruction programmed to eradicate you.

And avoiding estrogen replacement, as some pundits recommend, could do more harm than good.

The analysis I have prepared on breast cancer and hormones reaches a number of important conclusions:

- The overall evidence in the research literature says that estrogens—either natural estrogen or the standard patented, chemicalized estrogen substitutes (ERT)—do not increase the risk of aggressive breast cancer.
- There is evidence that estrogen use decreases mortality from breast cancer.
- There is conflicting evidence regarding breast cancer risk and the combined use of Premarin and Provera, the standard hormonal replacement (HRT) prescription. Some researchers say the combination increases risk while others say it decreases risk.
- There is evidence that progesterone has a strong protective effect against cancer.

The term *estrogen replacement therapy (ERT)* in contemporary medical practice does not refer to any natural balance of estrogen compounds. It refers to the patented pills, patches, or other forms of prescriptions containing certain components of your own estrogen or add-ons that make them unnatural to your body. Premarin is the most commonly used ERT prescription. The reports on estrogen and breast cancer you hear about relate to the patented, chemicalized pharmaceutical substitutes that are not the same as your own estrogen.

The term hormone replacement therapy (HRT) refers to combinations of these estrogen formulations along with a progestin accompaniment, mainly Provera, the pharmaceutical proxy for progesterone. Again, progestins are not progesterone—they are drugs.

In the history of "hormonal" therapy in the United States, women were first given estrogens, and primarily Premarin. In the mid-1970s, reports surfaced showing an increased incidence of endometrial cancer. This effect was attributed to using pharmaceutical estrogen alone. The whole pharmaceutical research focus then turned to protection of the uterus. Out of this effort emerged the development of progestins, including Provera, to counteract the effect of estrogen.

I have divided my analysis of breast cancer and hormones into five sections:

- Premarin (estrogen) alone—ERT.
- Premarin and Provera—HRT.
- HRT for patients with breast cancer.
- Natural estrogen and natural progesterone.
- Progesterone deficiency.

Premarin (Estrogen) Alone—ERT

In 1996, the American Cancer Society's research department reported a study of 442,000 menopausal women that evaluated the effect of estrogen use on breast cancer. After nine years of follow-up, 1,469 breast cancer deaths occurred in this group. None of the women had a diagnosis of cancer at the outset of the study period. The review of medical records found a *significant 16 percent decrease in the risk of fatal breast cancer* for the women who used ERT compared to nonusers.

Against the hysteria being raised about estrogen we need to look at the basic question: are more women dying from breast cancer because they take estrogen? This large study says no. Women using Premarin alone had a reduced risk of dying from breast cancer. Moreover, the researchers found no discernible trend of increased risk connected to length of use.

The data here also reinforce the findings of other studies about the nature of particular breast tumors. The research says clearly that women on ERT who develop breast cancer have a more benign, less aggressive, and less deadly type of cancer compared to non-ERT users.

In other words, if you develop cancer at all you are more likely to have a milder form of the disease when you take Premarin.

I have found six different studies that support this important distinction.

Some medical critics question the validity of these studies showing decreased breast cancer deaths among hormone users. The critics say that such women receive better medical supervision, and thus their tumors would be detected and treated earlier. This argument is illogical. All the data collected on ERT and the benefits of mammography demonstrate that estrogen treatment renders mammographic diagnosis less effective. Estrogen creates breast tissue that is more dense, as in a woman's younger years when the level of the hormone is higher. In many cases, the presence of denser tissue reduces the ability of radiologists to detect early tumors. So the claim is unsound that women who take estrogen have a lowered risk of breast cancer death because of early diagnosis. It is interesting to point out that *despite* the reduced mammographic effectiveness for ERT users, there is still a decreased risk of death from breast cancer.

A 1991 study reported in a Dutch medical journal described how the use of an estradiol (E2) implant under the skin decreased the incidence of breast cancer by 30 percent among women who had undergone hysterectomies. This method releases a constant supply of estradiol to the body. Estradiol, you will remember, is one of the three estrogen compounds.

Premarin and Provera — HRT

From 1975 to 1981, a large group (5,000 plus) of menopausal women were monitored at Lackland Air Force Base's Wilford Hall Medical Center in Texas. During this time, 256 women in the group were treated for breast cancer.

An analysis of hormone use among these women revealed the following statistics:

- Non-hormone users were found to have a breast cancer incidence equivalent to 342 per 100,000.
- Women who took Premarin alone (ERT) had an incidence of 141 per 100,000.

- Women who took Premarin with Provera, the usual hormonal replacement therapy (HRT) combination, had the lowest incidence by far—67 per 100,000.
- Nonusers who developed breast cancer were more likely to die from the condition than hormonal therapy patients, and also to experience increased metastasis to the axillary lymph nodes.

In 1999, R. Don Gambrell Jr., a leading breast cancer researcher who headed the study at Wilford Hall, reported further details on the fate of this same group of women. He found that now, with an additional nine to eighteen years of monitoring, 51 percent of the non-hormone users who developed breast cancer had died (85 out of 163) from the disease. Of the hormone users, 30 percent had passed away (19 out of 63).

According to Gambrell, the "most consistent, statistically significant decreased risk of breast cancer" was among the combined estrogen-progestin users.

In a review of the research provided to the author by Gambrell, four major studies evaluating combined therapy have determined a significant decrease of breast cancer risk when compared to non-hormone users or placebo-treated controls. Two of these studies involve twenty and twenty-two years of follow-up respectively. In the twenty-two-year study, not a single case of breast cancer developed among the 116 hormone therapy patients. Six cases of the disease developed among the fifty-two women who did not use hormones.

Recent studies from Sweden, Denmark, and the National Cancer Institute found a "nonsignificantly increased risk" of breast cancer among HRT patients, Gambrell pointed out. The Danish study involved only five years of observation. The Swedish study was based on only ten patients, and after an additional four years of monitoring, the researchers reported that the minor risk factor became even smaller.

In the widely publicized National Cancer Institute study, reported in the *Journal of the American Medical Association* in January 2000, only 4 percent of the 2,082 breast cancer patients used HRT. Among this group there was a statistically insignificant risk for breast cancer, Gambrell said.

However, in another recent study published in the February 2000 issue of the *Journal of the National Cancer Institute,* researchers at the University of Southern California found that the addition of a progestin to hormonal replacement therapy "enhances markedly the risk of breast cancer relative to estrogen use alone." A significant finding in the study connected a higher intake of Provera with an increased risk of breast cancer.

The inclusion of progestins into the breast cancer equation have produced conflicting evidence. When we step back from the confusion, we are still left with the disturbing facts that progestins such as Provera have serious negative effects on the cardiovascular system and take away the excellent benefits of estrogen. Clinically, I have observed how these drugs also upset the minds of women and cause anxiety. Compare this to the calming effect of natural progesterone.

Personally, I cannot understand the rationality of pouring questionable progestin drugs into women while a nondamaging and protective option is available, yet ignored. That option is natural progesterone.

HRT for Patients with Breast Cancer

I found nine studies involving HRT for patients with breast cancer. This conventional approach utilizes Premarin and Provera.

Most of the studies involve five years of follow-up or less. Yet each one of them demonstrated a decreased incidence of disease recurrence.

In a longer study, Jennifer Dew, M.D., an Australian physician at the Royal Hospital for Women in New South Wales, compared two groups of 167 women with a history of breast cancer. One group used hormonal therapy to relieve discomfort associated with menopause—90 percent of them took continuous progestin with estrogen drugs; the remainder took estrogen drugs only. The control group of women took no hormones at all.

After seven years of follow-up, the user group had a 9.6 percent recurrence of cancer, just under half the incidence (18.5 percent) of nonusers.

The researchers suggested that the combined, continuous therapy may help block tumor formation.

Natural Estrogen and Natural Progesterone

Unfortunately, there is no research information on the long-term use of natural estrogen and progesterone in hormonal replacement therapy related to breast cancer. Yet two million years of evolution and all the information available in physiology books suggest that the best solution is to copy our body's own hormonal protocol:

Natural estrogen + Natural progesterone = Protection

Progesterone Deficiency

There are four studies in the medical literature associating a *deficiency of progesterone* with an increased risk of breast cancer.

In a 1981 issue of the *American Journal of Epidemiology*, Linda Cowan and colleagues at Johns Hopkins University reported on the relationship of naturally occurring progesterone and cancer during perimenopause. They studied a thousand women, originally evaluated and treated for infertility from 1945 to 1965, monitoring them until 1978 to determine the incidence of breast cancer. They divided the women into two groups according to the cause of infertility: (1) a progesterone deficiency group, and (2) a group with normal progesterone and non–hormone based infertility.

The researchers found that progesterone exerts a strong preventive effect against cancer. The group with normal levels of progesterone had a fivefold lower risk of developing premenopausal breast cancer, and a tenfold lower risk of dying from any type of cancer, compared to the women with a hormone deficiency.

In a 1983 study reported in the *Journal of the American Medical Association* researchers found an increased risk associated with chronic anovulation, a term meaning lack of ovulation. This is usually caused by a progesterone deficiency.

I believe these studies add another major clue to our understanding of how cancer develops. We can see that progesterone, with all its protective benefits to the body, is a critical element in the fight against cancer.

The medical literature also includes several interesting studies showing that young women who undergo mastectomies for breast cancer have a much better survival rate and recurrence-free prognosis when the surgery is performed during the luteal phase of the menstrual cycle. This is the time of the month when the body produces the most progesterone. Because of the potential for saving lives and preventing recurrences, this area of research should be vigorously pursued.

What Is Missing from the Research

The glaring omission from all the research is the exclusion of natural hormones into the consideration of prevention and therapeutic approaches to breast cancer.

Pharmaceutical products have become the research and clinical standards. The large pharmaceutical companies have the financial resources to pay for the huge research, development, and marketing costs associated with medical drugs. They research a natural substance, such as a hormone, and then alter it or add to it, to make it different. The changed product is patented, that is, given legal protection against another company copying it.

Obviously a pharmaceutical company must protect its investment—I understand that. But the medical authorities should not allow these particular products to be misrepresented as hormones. They are drugs. If they were to be called what they are—drugs, and not hormones—you would not be so confused. You wouldn't think that the medical reports are talking about your own hormones.

Research on natural hormones is sorely lacking. There is little data to give us useful comparisons for this very promising option. Where is the money to come from? Companies will not invest the many millions of dollars needed to obtain medical use approval for a natural compound that anybody can copy.

The reality is sad, particularly as it relates to cancer. Research on hormone replacement therapy and cancer is really research on drugs and cancer. To say they are studies on hormones is a misrepresentation. It's as if you claim to investigate the effect of liquid intake on athletic performance and use alcohol instead of water.

The cancer research community does women a great injustice by continuing to ignore natural hormones. The financial interests of companies should not take priority over the welfare of half the population.

The restoration of natural hormonal balance in the body is missing from contemporary HRT. Human evolution gives us the perspective with which to create healthier and vital lives even as we live longer than we ever have before. Hopefully, open-minded clinicians and open-minded patients looking for safe and effective alternatives will help influence the medical community's one-sided approach to hormonal replacement.

More on the Estrogen Connection

Many women are fearful of fertility treatments because the drugs used over a two-week period dramatically increase the levels of estrogens in the body. Yet for the nine months of pregnancy, the body produces much more estrogen. The levels of aggressive estrogens—estrone and estradiol—increase four times or more than normal. And we know that full-term pregnancy is associated with a decreased incidence of breast cancer.

Why is this? Because the elevation of aggressive estrogens is overshadowed by an even more significant rise in protective estriol and progesterone. This is nature's two-million-year-old protection formula.

In Western societies, a historical breakaway from the norm of multiple childbirth has taken place in the twentieth century. With this departure from the age-old reproductive pattern, the modern woman has lost the same degree of hormonal protection her antecedents had during many cycles of pregnancy and breast-feeding.

If estrogen were the great villain of breast cancer we would have expected to see an overnight surge of the disease in the very first generations of Western women who broke with the age-old reproductive tradition. These are the great-grandmothers, grandmothers, and mothers of my generation who generally delivered far fewer children. You now had massive numbers of women with much of their progesterone protection gone. They produced progesterone for only half of their monthly cycle in their fertile years, and little or none later in life.

Despite the unprecedented emergence of widespread estrogen dominance that resulted, there was no sudden epidemic of breast cancer in these generations. It is with the women of my wife's generation that we see the incidence of breast cancer take an alarming upturn.

The incidence of breast cancer has doubled since 1950 in the United States. In Asia there is now an explosion of breast cancer.

What is going on? What has changed? Why are women today so vulnerable? What is behind the increase in breast cancer?

According to breast cancer authority R. Don Gambrell Jr., of the Medical College of Georgia, *there are at least seventy studies on estrogen therapy showing that even unopposed estrogens do not increase the risk of dying from breast cancer.*

So why do you hear about estrogen being "on trial" or linked to breast cancer?

For the answer, we need to take a brief excursion into the cellular world of breast tissue and consider some of the latest research concepts.

Imagine that we take a quantity of estradiol (E2), one of the three estrogen compounds produced in the human body, and rub it on the breasts. Estradiol, you will remember, is one of the so-called aggressive estrogens.

What happens? The estradiol is absorbed into the tissue and accelerates the natural replication of cells. In other words, it will cause a proliferation of the normal cells in the breasts.

It is safe to say that by itself, estradiol will not cause cancer. However, if cancer cells are present in the tissue, the estrogen will stimulate them to grow faster as well. Yet the presence of estrogen seems to influence the development of the growth into a less aggressive and more benign form. We refer to this as a "well differentiated tumor."

In order for a cell to turn cancerous, the DNA, that is, the genetic command post of the cell that governs its function, must become mutated in some way. This occurs when estrone and estradiol, the aggressive forms of estrogen, enter into breast cells where they are metabolized and converted into different by-products or metabolites. They go by the names of 2-catechol estrone, 4-catechol estrone, and 16-alpha-hydroxyestrone.

Researchers agree that 2-catechol estrone is a benign substance. *Not only benign, it is also protective.* The higher the level of this compound the lower the incidence of breast cancer.

On the other hand, the other two compounds have been identified as initiators of the cancer process. They can damage DNA and trigger mutation leading to the development of cancer. This sequence is believed by researchers to be indeed involved in the formation of many forms of cancer, in both women and men (estrogen is also produced by men). Breast, brain, ovarian, and prostate cancer are examples. Research conducted at the University of Nebraska has found extra high levels of 4-catechol compounds in patients with breast cancer.

The body, as you know, is a remarkable organism with powerful check-and-balance systems. It has the ability to keep this potentially harmful estrogen conversion process in check through a network of deactivating and repair enzymes.

These protective agents are called catechol 0 methyl transferase, COMT for short. The blocking action they perform is just one small part of a remarkable enzyme system constantly at work in the trillions of cells in your body that converts substances into other substances. The process is called methylation.

In this case, if the process works well, it protects you against cellular mutation and the development of cancer cells. If methylation is defective for some reason, the level of protection suffers. University of Nebraska researchers also found that women with breast cancer were lacking in COMT, the protective enzyme. And at Johns Hopkins University, research suggests that low COMT can contribute to the menopausal development of breast cancer in many women.

You might wonder what causes a lack of COMT. Here I need to introduce another biochemical player into the equation. It's homocysteine, an amino acid known to trigger arterial plaque and blood clot formation when it reaches toxic levels in the body. High homocysteine is an indicator of a lack of methylation, and thus has a role in promoting cancer. Homocysteine becomes elevated as a result of deficiency in B vitamins (vitamin B_6, B_{12}, and folic acid). Vegetables and whole grains are a rich source of these vitamins. Sugary, processed foods deplete the body of these vitamins. So there is an important nutritional connection here.

Measuring the homocysteine level in your blood is a good way to determine both your methylation ability and your vascular health. In a moment I will discuss how you can lower high homocysteine, increase COMT, and promote methylation with nutritional supplements.

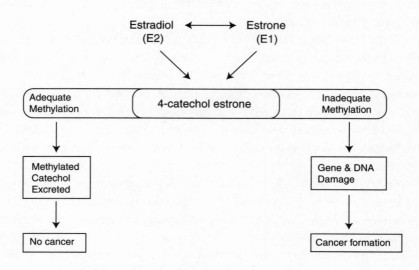

DEPICTION OF CANCER FORMATION SEQUENCE

Cancer and the Toxic Environment

Any consideration of the dramatic rise in breast cancer must include a major factor that tends to be ignored—environmental toxins. We live in a very toxic world. Contaminants continually enter our bodies through the food, water, and air that sustain us. It is not coincidental that the dramatic rise of cancer in the world has occurred at a time of unparalleled proliferation of synthetic chemicals and toxins.

I don't consider myself an environmental fanatic, and this book is not meant to be a crusade about global toxicity. I am grateful for the many comforts and advances that chemical technology has brought us, but as a physician I am concerned about the harm that this powerful technology has unleashed as well.

There are some 75,000 chemicals in industrial and commercial use. Only a tiny percentage has been tested for safety. How many of these are carcinogenic no one knows. But experts like Samuel Epstein of the University of

Chicago believe that the proliferation of chemicals has created unprecedented pollutants and carcinogens in the environment that are primary contributors to the cancer epidemic.

Studies have linked increased breast cancer in women exposed to certain chemicals in industrial work or even from living near toxic waste dumps.

In 1993, researchers at the U.S. Department of Health and Human Services published a report hypothesizing that certain chemicals, herbicides, and pharmaceuticals could promote the cellular mutation leading to breast cancer. According to Devra Lee Davis, the chief author of the report and now an epidemiologist at the World Resources Institute, many of these compounds, such as those in plastics, fuels, and pesticides, appear to increase the risk of breast cancer.

These substances tend to settle in fatty tissue, such as breast tissue, where they accumulate and create genetic damage. Even minute amounts of some of these substances can trigger cancer cells.

One of the most notorious chemicals is dioxin, a family of toxic substances produced in many industrial processes involving chlorine or chlorine-based chemicals. PVC plastics, chlorinated solvents, chlorinated pesticides, and chlorine bleached paper are leading causes of dioxin release into the environment and food supply.

We are all exposed to significant amounts of dioxin and related pollutants. Wildlife populations, including fish, birds, and marine mammals, have been already severely affected by dioxin. The U.S. Environmental Protection Agency has warned that this contaminant poses a long-term threat to health.

A number of studies have shown that dioxin significantly increases the production of P450 1B1, an enzyme that converts estrogen into the dangerous 4-catechol form. This may be a missing clue as to how the toxic environment may contribute to an increased risk of breast cancer.

Some patients have asked me about dioxin in tampons. I checked into this and learned that tampons are made of cotton, rayon, or blends of both materials. Rayon is manufactured from cellulose fibers processed from wood pulp. At one time, chlorine compounds were used to bleach the wood pulp and thus were a potential source of trace amounts of dioxin.

According to the Food and Drug Administration (FDA), current manufacturing methods emphasize the reduction of dioxin levels. Moreover, producers are required to routinely monitor dioxin.

"Because of decades of pollution, dioxin can be found in the air, water, and ground," says the FDA. "Therefore, while the methods used for manufacturing tampons today are considered to be dioxin-free processes, traces of dioxin may still be present in the cotton or wood pulp raw materials used to make tampons. Thus, there may be trace amounts of dioxin present from environmental sources in cotton, rayon, or rayon/cotton tampons."

The FDA's risk assessment indicates that this exposure is "many times less than normally present in the body from other environmental sources, so small that any risk of adverse health effects is considered negligible."

I am more concerned about the level of dioxins and similar compounds into our food supply. Dioxin expert Arnold Schecter, of the State University Health Science Center in Binghamton, New York, has collected samples of typical food around the United States and found trace amounts that far exceed many government regulations. Dioxin levels are highest in fatty foods.

Diet and Cancer

Researchers have found that obesity is related to an increased risk of cancer, including breast cancer. Obese women have a lower level of the 2-catechol estrogen (the good metabolite of estrogen) when compared to long-distance runners. Fat cells in the body, it turns out, secrete an enzyme that inhibits the transformation of estradiol and estrone to 2-catechol estrone.

Where do the fat cells come from? Is it from eating a lot of fat in the diet? High fat intake has been hypothesized for many years as an important risk factor for breast cancer. But research is equivocal on the subject. Some investigators say it is important, while others say that decreasing fat intake does not decrease the risk.

After reading considerable research and hearing many of the leading experts I believe that certain fats indeed contribute to cancer. I have in mind chemicalized, highly processed fats, such as hydrogenated and partially hydrogenated oils that give longer shelf life to food products. These types of fats promote free radical activity in the body, a major cause of disease and accelerated aging. However, it is beyond the scope of this book to explore this complex issue.

A recent Italian study shed light on what is being increasingly seen as a new culprit—high carbohydrate intake. The study compared menopausal women with breast cancer to women without the disease. The researchers looked at dietary intake and concluded that high intake of refined bread and pasta led to an increase of cancer risk. Olive and seed oils were found to be protective.

The Italian eating style offers a good model for such studies. Italians tend to eat a more limited diet in comparison to Americans, who choose many different types of food.

The study dramatizes an ignored metabolic reality: your body converts carbohydrates into body fat more readily than it does the fat you eat. *It's a fact that you don't lose weight by cutting out fat, but by cutting down on carbohydrates.*

In our society we eat too many carbohydrates. We load up on sugary foods, chips, cookies, cake, pasta and bread, and carbohydrates of all types. The body breaks down carbohydrates into a sugar called glucose. After a meal or snack, the hormone insulin is released by the pancreas to move glucose into the cells for conversion into energy. But insulin also promotes fat storage as well. The greater the amount of insulin produced by the body, in answer to increased carbohydrate consumption, the greater the amount of fat that is stored. High insulin is also associated with increased free radical damage, a leading contributor to disease.

Women with breast cancer have been told to eat low-fat diets. It seems to me they should be eating fewer carbohydrates instead, and step up their protein and fresh vegetable intake. That may be the best way to avoid adulthood weight gain, which may include a significant reduction in the risk of menopausal breast cancer.

Ideas for Cancer Prevention

Cancer is a complicated issue without simple answers and magic bullets. We live in a complicated world where health is impacted by our own actions as well as by many elements beyond our control. Prevention is the name of the game, and for breast cancer I believe it starts with progesterone.

The Natural Progesterone Weapon

I can't emphasize progesterone enough. In part three I explained the many ways that your own progesterone contributes to health in general and protection against cancer specifically. As a hormone replacement strategy, natural progesterone is a natural choice for prevention. It strengthens the immune system and blocks estrogen dominance.

At least one study has shown that a 10 percent progesterone cream applied to the breasts can powerfully reduce the tendency of breast cells to replicate fast.

Recent laboratory experiments conducted by T. S. Wiley and Bent Formby, at the Sansum Medical Research Institute in Santa Barbara, indicate that a relatively high level of progesterone, similar to that present during the third trimester of pregnancy, exerts a strong antiproliferative effect on breast cancer cells.

Unfortunately, not a single study on HRT and breast cancer involves natural progesterone. There is no research on the natural hormone but hundreds on the patented, chemicalized hormonal substitutes. This is a sad testimony. If the health of citizens is the ultimate concern, it doesn't make sense to limit research to pharmaceuticals alone and ignore the potential of natural hormones.

I am also concerned about advertising claims for low-potency progesterone creams as a strategy against breast cancer. Even if they are natural, there is no evidence that they are sufficiently strong enough to provide systemic or local protection.

The Estriol Weapon

Since the 1970s, a limited number of studies have found that estriol (E3), one of the three estrogen compounds in the body, is a highly protective substance. Unlike its estrone (E1) and estradiol (E2) sister compounds, it appears to have little or no ability to convert into the destructive estrogen metabolites that ignite cellular mutation.

In a laboratory experiment conducted two decades ago, H. M. Lemon, M.D., of the University of Nebraska Medical Center, found that young female rats exposed to cancer-causing radiation or strong chemicals actually developed 80 percent fewer mammary malignancies if they were given estriol beforehand.

Lemon also reported that clinical experience with oral estriol therapy for menopausal women "has indicated little hazard of cancer development."

Why isn't estriol studied for inclusion in hormonal replacement therapy? Could we achieve a dramatic reduction in breast cancer by supplementing teenage girls with estriol?

We also need studies to give us good statistical data on the benefits of estriol and how much we should use in proportion to estrone and estradiol.

Estriol is not in the female body by mistake. It is the most abundant of the estrogen compounds in your body. And during pregnancy, the level of estriol soars well beyond the surge of estrone or estradiol, or even progesterone.

In a 1987 article in the medical journal *Cancer,* Lemon suggested that the physiologic maturation of breast tissue characteristic of pregnancy might be simulated by the use of estriol for young women who are barren. This might "increase durable resistance" against tumor formation, he said.

In Europe, estriol has long been administered to many women for relief of menopausal symptoms.

I prescribe estriol alone to patients with a history of breast cancer who do not want to use estradiol. But in general I believe that natural estrogen replacement, which includes all three estrogen compounds, is the best way to go for hormonal balance. That's what evolution has given to women. That's what I recommend to my patients. That's what I recommend to you.

Reducing Exposure to Environmental Toxins

Many environmental chemicals enter the body and become stored in fat cells, including the cells of the breast. There they build up, interfere with healthy cellular function, and prime the cells for disease.

Unfortunately, there is often little you can do about global pollutants such as dioxin, but you can take steps to detoxify your immediate surroundings by using natural, nontoxic detergents, hair sprays, carpet cleansers, etc. You do have choices.

I recommend two excellent books that can give you numerous practical tips:

* *Clean House, Clean Plane: Clean Your House for Pennies a Day the Safe, Nontoxic Way,* by Karen Logan (Pocket Books, 1997).
* *Home Safe Home: Protecting Yourself and Your Family from Everyday Toxins and Harmful Household Products,* by Debra Lynn Dadd (Putnam Publishing Group, 1997). Miss Dadd also has an information-packed Internet Web site: www.dld123.com.

I regard all these toxins as health threats. They have the potential to affect you on a short-term or long-term basis. I think we all need to do whatever we can to cut down exposure.

The Food Weapon

Regarding diet, there is no data showing that high carbohydrate and low fat intake, or avoiding meat, reduces cancer. I have seen considerable data, however, indicating that maintaining a low percentage of body fat might decrease the incidence of breast cancer. The way I interpret the most current expertise is that a diet comprising about 30 percent protein, 30 percent fat, and 40 percent carbohydrates may be the most effective way to accomplish this.

As a society, we are obsessed with how much fat, carbs, and protein we should eat. We tend to forget about quality and purity. Personally, I try to eat as much organic food as possible so as to cut down on the residual pesticides, herbicides, and other chemical toxins used in commercial food production that have no business in our bodies.

I realize that organic is more expensive than "regular" food. But if we use our food budget more wisely to buy organic food instead and eliminate some of the junk food and less wholesome choices, we would probably be healthier. For sure, anyone with a serious illness such as cancer should be eating food of as high a quality as possible.

I recommend frequent servings of broccoli, cabbage, Brussels sprouts, and cauliflower. They may not be your favorite foods but this family of vegetables contains a naturally occurring substance you should know about—indole-3-carbinol. We call it I3C for short.

Research by H. Leon Bradlow and colleagues at the Strang Cancer Research Laboratory in New York have repeatedly shown that this phytonutrient powerfully boosts the cellular conversion of estrogen into the 2-catechol form—in other words, the good metabolite of estrogen. At the same time it sharply decreases activity leading to the carcinogenic 4-catechol formation. This antitumor activity has been demonstrated in both animal and human studies.

Doesn't it make more sense to use something like I3C than tamoxifen, a primary drug prescribed to women with breast cancer or a high risk of developing it? Tamoxifen is an antiestrogen agent.

But Tamoxifen is clearly a questionable drug. While it may protect against breast cancer, it has multiple undesirable effects on the body:

1. It promotes uterine cancer.
2. It significantly increases blood clot formation and the risk of life-threatening pulmonary embolisms.
3. It can lead to "toxicity" of the eye and possibly increase the susceptibility to cataracts when used long term.

Tamoxifen's protection from breast cancer lasts only *on average* five years. According to research, if it is taken longer it becomes cancer causing! What about the women for whom it becomes carcinogenic before five years?

Moreover, a certain gene called HER-2 plays a pivotal role in an aggressive type of tumor that can be found in about 10 percent of breast cancer cases. Tamoxifen may accelerate the activity of this gene and speed tumor growth in these cases.

As a taxpayer, I would like to propose an idea to the government. When federal funds are used to support cancer drug research, give the project a few extra dollars to test natural substances as well, such as I3C. Instead of a controlled double blind, for instance, do a triple-blind study. Test the drug, the natural substance, and the placebo. Or include long-term studies with users of natural substances and not just drugs. That gives taxpayers a real return for the research we subsidize. With the devastating incidence of cancer in our society, how can our leaders declare a war on cancer without testing all the weapons?

The Supplement Weapon

At the top of the list is indole-3-carbinol. I suggest 400 milligrams a day. You can buy I3C at health food stores. I recommend this supplement to all my patients, and particularly if they have been taking the birth control pill or using chemicalized HRT for many years, have a family history of breast cancer, or have been found to be in a situation of estrogen dominance.

If you already take vitamin and mineral supplements, be sure to include or add the following in your program:

- Vitamin B$_6$
- Vitamin B$_{12}$
- Folic acid
- SAM-e
- Trimethylglycine

Each of these nutritional factors is important to promote methylation in the body. This is the process I described earlier that conducts basic enzymatic and genetic transformations in the cells. In our discussion of breast cancer we have seen how proper methylation inhibits the progression of 4-catechol estrone into cancer.

SAM-e, short for S-adenosylmethionine, is the active form of the amino acid methionine. It is required in virtually every methylation process in the body.

A deficiency of vitamins B$_6$, B$_{12}$, and folic acid, all members of the B complex family, has been shown to reduce the availability of SAM-e in the body. Aging has also been shown to decrease the level of SAM-e. So it is important to supplement these factors.

A low level of the B vitamins is the main cause of elevated homocysteine. High homocysteine, as I mentioned earlier, contributes to blood vessel disease and cancer.

Trimethylglycine, or TMG, is a quasi-vitamin that helps normalize defective amino acid metabolism, and particularly in patients who have high homocysteine unresponsive to vitamin B$_6$ supplementation. It helps to "remethylate" homocysteine, meaning that it converts homocysteine to methionine for use in the body. TMG is also a powerful antioxidant.

I also recommend a number of potent antioxidants to my patients:

- Lycopene
- Co-enzyme Q10
- Melatonin

Antioxidants are important neutralizers of free radical activity in the body. Free radicals are like renegade molecular fragments typically generated by toxins and chemicals. If the body's defense system doesn't contain them, they inflict widespread damage by inhibiting normal methylation activities. This results in tissue damage, disease, and accelerated aging.

According to research reported in the medical literature, lycopene, co-enzyme Q10, and melatonin provide a protective effect against breast cancer.

All the supplements I have mentioned here are available in health food stores.

A Final Word

Don't let anybody scare you about cancer and your own hormones.

Estrogen is not causing the epidemic in breast cancer. It is more likely the lack of natural progesterone, plus other risk factors such as the proliferation of chemicals that generate cell mutations.

The studies show that estrogens are not associated with increased mortality from breast cancer. The variety of progestins available may or may not increase the incidence of breast cancer, depending on which study you consider. However, there are many serious problems with progestins.

Progesterone offers natural protection against cancer.

Try to align your hormonal replacement therapy choices with nature's own compounds. Choose a natural estrogen hormone such as Tri-Est that contains all three estrogens: estrone, estradiol, and estriol.

Avoid estrogen dominance, which can cause problems. You can avoid estrogen dominance by using progesterone. Progesterone means protection and prevention.

Whatever your choices, there is no need to be confused or afraid.

24

The Future of Hormone Therapy

In my practice I have seen the magnificent results of natural hormone therapy. I have seen it work with menopausal, perimenopausal, and younger women. I have seen it turn back the biological clock of older women, giving them restored energy, clarity, positivity, sensuality, and health. I have seen it prevent younger women from imbalances and deficiencies that make them feel, act, and look much older.

What is really fascinating for me as a physician is that I have seen thousands of women adopt this method and eagerly work with it as an empowerment tool. In the process, they learn intimately how their bodies work, how they can take control and no longer be a victim of hormonal fluctuations, and how to raise themselves in the process to a higher level of functioning.

I am troubled by the direction of hormonal replacement therapy. When I read the medical literature or hear experts at medical conferences speak about "what's in the pipeline" it is clear that the direction is a continued emphasis on chemicalized hormonal substitutes. I have yet in my medical career to come across a substitute that didn't create some side effect.

I hear the experts talk about these drugs in impersonal, technical terms. They will speak, for instance, about bone density improvement. Scientists like to measure things, and I can appreciate that. And for sure, as four thousand women in North America reach menopause every day, they are concerned about osteoporosis.

But women are concerned about much more than their bones. They are obviously concerned about breast cancer and heart disease. They are also concerned about things that scientists can't measure. My patients are concerned about fatigue, mental clarity and memory, anxiety, depression, tender breasts, and the inability to fall asleep. They are concerned about how they look, feel, and think.

I don't hear the experts talking about these things. Can chemicalized hormonal substitutes address all these concerns? Or do they eliminate one symptom and create a new one?

Unfortunately, the trend is moving *away* from what is natural to what is pharmaceutical. It's moving away from nature, away from a woman's own precise and unique composition of hormones, and away from natural compounds that have been part of the biochemical symphony of her body since time immemorial.

Are we pharmaceutical beings or natural beings?

If we take these drugs maybe we will create women with strong bones but who are depressed, without spirit, energy, and mental clarity.

This book was written in order to help bring the potential of natural hormones to the attention of women. I see natural hormones as an option promising balance and rescue for a contemporary practice of hormonal replacement therapy beset with imbalance, confusion, and lack of compliance. Natural hormones have the potential to transform disorder into order.

The current consumer interest in natural healing has caused a revolution within the medical establishment. More and more patients are demanding natural options. They want more than just another version of drug X. In response, physicians are learning more about natural healing and offering new approaches.

Many more women than men seek medical help. Perhaps this female force of patients can create the same consumer pressure for natural hormonal therapy. Why shouldn't it be offered?

At some future date, I believe that medical technology will develop a computerized multihormone patch that a woman can use for a lifetime. Applied to the skin, it will be capable of measuring key hormonal levels in the body and responding with the exact transdermal replacement of hormones to maintain optimum physiological function.

Such a patch would be used initially when a woman is in her peak hormonal years to "load" the memory system with data regarding her individual optimum hormone profile. Later, as she ages and her hormone levels decline, the device will refer to its stored hormonal data and replace back into the system the appropriate replacement quantities of hormones to maintain balance and youthfulness.

I look forward to such technology, but please let the technology include natural hormones.

Let us use our immeasurable creativity to maximize the benefits instead of replacing old symptoms with new side effects.

I will be most happy to allow a computer to conduct the symphony of hormones and bring us into a new era of antiaging and health possibilities.

Appendix A

Where to Buy Natural Hormones

Compounding pharmacies are the most reliable source for all the natural hormones described in this book. They are the only source for estrogen, progesterone, and testosterone that require prescriptions.

Retail outlets, such as health food stores, drugstores, and Internet vendors, carry the following products that require no prescription:

- Low-potency progesterone creams
- DHEA
- Pregnenolone
- Melatonin
- Human growth hormone substitutes.

Compounding pharmacies customize drugs, nutritional supplements, and natural hormones for physicians and patients. The licensed pharmacists who work at compounding pharmacies mix, assemble, package, and label these preparations using high-quality, government-approved raw chemicals, powders, and natural substances.

Some compounding pharmacies are part of drugstores where the usual commercial array of medications and household hygiene products are sold. Others specialize in only compounding activities. By comparison, the regular commercial pharmacy you are familiar with primarily dispenses an already manufactured form of a particular drug or medication.

In chapter 4, I made some suggestions about how to approach your physician if he or she is not familiar with natural hormones or may be part of a health plan that does not cover these preparations.

If your doctor won't write you a prescription, you may want to contact a compounding pharmacy and ask for the names of physicians in your area who use natural hormones. Such health professionals are limited to medical doctors, osteopathic doctors, and (in some states) naturopaths.

The American Academy of Anti-Aging Medicine is another good source for the names of doctors who often treat patients with natural hormones. You can write the organization at 1341 W. Fullerton, Suite 111, Chicago IL 60614, or call 773-528-4333, or find it on the Internet at www.worldhealth.net.

Prescriptions are called or faxed to the compounding pharmacy. Start with a one-month supply. Once you have become familiar with dosage and your individual needs, you may want your physician to order a larger supply, such as for three months.

Insurance companies and health plans are increasingly covering natural hormone prescriptions. Check with your health plan provider. Some plans may only reimburse you for one month at a time. Some plans may contract with specific compounding pharmacies.

As a courtesy, and where applicable, some pharmacies may bill the insurance carrier. You should be prepared, however, to pay for the prescription with a credit card or check.

Compounding pharmacies can fill your prescriptions as a cream, gel, pill, sublingual drop, or suppository. Follow my guidelines in the book, and with your physician select the best form for your particular situation. If you are using multiple hormones, wait until you are familiar with their individual effects before you opt to combine them in one product. Take them separately until then.

When you are ready, the compounding pharmacist can combine hormones for you in whichever form you choose and even flavor it if you so desire. Creams and gels are accompanied with applicators that help you measure out a precise amount of the hormone preparation.

If you have special concerns, such as a sensitivity to a substance used in the natural hormone preparation, speak directly to a pharmacist.

If you are allergic to soy, it is very unlikely you will experience a reaction to a natural hormone made from soy. That's because the original plant material has passed through multiple chemical processes en route to its ultimate transformation into the pure hormone. There is essentially no soy left in the pure hormonal powder. Nevertheless, if you have a question, speak to the pharmacist.

Once an order is filled it is shipped directly to the patient.

Over the years I have worked closely with two first-class compounding pharmacies:

Kronos Compounding Pharmacy
3675 South Rainbow
Las Vegas, NV 89103
(800) 723-7455
Fax: (800) 238-8239

Women's International Pharmacy (two locations)
5708 Monona Drive   13925 W. Meeker Boulevard
Madison, WI 53716-3152   Sun City West, AZ 85375
(800) 279-5708
Fax: (800) 279-8011

The consistent quality of their prescriptions has been an important supportive factor in my ability to understand natural hormones and conduct accurate medical tests to monitor the hormones. In addition, the pharmacy staff has always been very courteous and responsive to my patients and their needs.

There are many excellent compounding pharmacies around the country that can also provide you and your physician with excellent service.

Keep the following in mind when you choose a compounding pharmacy: the chemical composition of each particular natural hormone is the same, no matter from which pharmacy it is obtained. However, the bases, such as the types of oils used as delivery mediums (carriers) for the hormones, may vary from pharmacy to pharmacy. This might affect the rate and amount of absorption and could possibly lead to results different from those I have described in the book. In such cases, your physician might have to change the dose you are using or consult with the pharmacist about changing a base ingredient in the prescription formula.

I should also point out that blood tests of hormone levels based on over-the-counter hormones may be unreliable. There are sometimes wide differences between potencies listed on product labels and actual contents. For the sake of guaranteed purity, I suggest to patients that they obtain their natural hormones—prescription items as well as nonprescription items—from a compounding pharmacy, or only purchase the highest-quality, best-known over-the-counter brands.

Appendix B

Beware of Hidden Hormones in Health Products

Georgia was three years into menopause. She had been following a standard hormonal replacement therapy with Premarin and Provera for some time when she was diagnosed with breast cancer. At the suggestion of her gynecologist, she stopped the hormones.

Georgia then made an appointment to see me. She was desperate for help. However, she refused to follow my recommendation to start a combined estriol (E3) and progesterone program that I knew would be protective for her. She would have nothing to do with any form of estrogen. I tried to help her with soy, black cohosh, and other herbal and nutritional supplements but was unable to make progress.

A few months later Georgia called my office. She was elated. She was feeling great and said she had "triumphed over conventional medicine."

"What are you taking?" I asked.

"I consulted with this great nutritionist and he gave me some herbs to take," she answered. "Not only did I get better, but my own natural hormones have returned. I have even started to bleed again."

"Well," I said, "over the years I have seen many menopausal patients who don't take hormones experience a spontaneous and temporary return of bleeding. But you should come back for an evaluation. I would like to see you."

If indeed she was having a spontaneous return of menstruation that could mean her body was producing estrogen without any progesterone to balance it out. This means unopposed estrogen, a situation that could increase her risk for cancer in the uterus.

I asked Georgia to come back and bring the herbal products she was using. When she showed them to me I recognized ingredients that included herbs and phytoestrogens. Such substances should not increase the estrogen level in the blood, and certainly not progesterone. Yet a blood test showed her estrogen level was high normal and her progesterone was low. At this stage of menopause, her estrogen and progesterone levels should have been extremely low.

I immediately suspected that there were hidden hormones among the herbs she was taking—namely a good deal of estrogen and a small amount of progesterone. Sure she was feeling good. She didn't know it but she was taking hormones, including estrogen, which she had earlier rejected.

I asked her to stop the product for a few days and then return for another blood test. In three days, her hormonal level had returned to a more typical menopausal picture. She had also regained the signs of estrogen deficiency.

I have seen many cases like Georgia's over the years, perhaps because I practice in an area where people are very much into natural healing. On numerous occasions patients have shown me supplements supposedly containing wild yam or soy extracts that they purchased from nutritionists or nonmedical health practitioners. In reality, they contained the real thing—progesterone or estrogen—and in potencies much higher than the over-the-counter limitation. Nutritionists, who are very knowledgeable about nutritional supplements, are not trained in endocrinology. They may have little understanding of the complexities of hormones and hormone balance.

Georgia, a woman with breast cancer, had refused to take estrogen, not even estriol, the most protective estrogen compound. Now she was led to believe she was taking herbs when in fact she was getting estrogen and progesterone.

I strongly condemn the illegal mislabeling and distribution of such products. I also condemn their use by unqualified practitioners. There is potential here to harm innocent patients, as well as give a bad name to the natural supplement industry and the community of ethical nutritionists.

If you are estrogen or progesterone deficient and you start using any natural supplement that suddenly eliminates your symptoms, do yourself a favor and have your blood estradiol (E2) and progesterone levels checked. An herbal product cannot increase your estradiol or progesterone values. If your levels are higher, you are taking hormones, not herbs.

Selected References

Adams, M. R., et al. "Medroxyprogesterone acetate antagonizes inhibitory effects of conjugatedequine estrogens on coronary artery atherosclerosis." *Arterioscler Thromb Vasc Biol,* January 1997, 17 (1): 217–21.

Antonijevic, Irina, et al. "Modulation of the sleep electroencephalogram by estrogen replacement in postmenopausal women." *American Journal of Obstetrics and Gynecology,* February 2000: 277.

Aparasu, R. R. "Visits to office-based physicians in the United States for medication-related morbidity." *Journal of the American Pharm Asso,* May-June 1999, 39 (3): 332–7.

Araneo, B., et al. "DHEAS as an effective vaccine adjuvant in elderly humans." *Annals of the New York Academy of Sciences,* 1995, 774: 232–48.

Arlt, W., et al. "Dehydroepiandrosterone replacement in women with adrenal insufficiency." *New England Journal of Medicine,* September 30, 1999, 341 (14): 1013–20.

Badwe, R. A., et al. "Timing of surgery during menstrual cycle and survival of premenopausal women with operable breast cancer." *Lancet,* 1991, 337: 1261–4.

———. "Timing of surgery with regard to the menstrual cycle in women with primary breast cancer." *Surgical Clinics of North America,* October 1999, 79 (5): 1047–59.

Baker, Valerie L. "Alternatives to oral estrogen replacement: Transdermal patches, percutaneous gels, vaginal creams and rings, implants and other methods of delivery." *Obstetrics and Gynecology Clinics of North America,* June 1994, 21 (2): 271–97.

Bailar, John C., and Gornik, Heather. "Cancer undefeated." *New England Journal of Medicine,* May 29, 1997, 336 (22): 1569–74.

Barrett-Connor, E., et al. "The epidemiology of DHEAS and cardiovascular disease." *Annals of the New York Academy of Sciences,* 1995, 774: 259–70.

————. "Endogenous levels of dehydroepiandrosterone sulfate, but not other sex hormones, are associated with depressed mood in older women: the Rancho Bernardo Study." *Journal of the American Geriatric Society,* June 1999, 47 (6): 685–91.

Bartsch, C., and Bartsch, H. "Melatonin in cancer patients and in tumor-bearing animals." *Advances in Exper Med Biol,* 1999, 467: 247–64.

Batt, Sharon, and Gross, Liza. "Cancer, Inc." *Sierra Magazine,* September/October 1999: 36.

Baulieu, E. E., et al. "Dehydroepiandrosterone (DHEA), DHEA sulfate, and aging: Contribution of the DHEAge Study to a sociobiomedical issue." *Proceedings of the National Academy of Sciences USA,* April 11, 2000, 97 (8): 4279–84.

Baum, A. L. "Selective serotonin-reuptake inhibitors in pregnancy and lactation." *Harvard Review of Psychiatry,* September 1996, 4 (3): 117–25.

Bilimoria, M. M., et al. "Estrogen replacement therapy and breast cancer: analysis of age of onset and tumor characteristics." *Annals of Surgical Oncology,* 1999, 6: 200–7

Bluming, A. Z., et al. "Hormone replacement therapy in women with previously treated primary breast cancer." *Proceedings of the Annual Meeting of the American Society of Clinical Oncology,* 1994, Abstract A137.

Bonnier, P., et al. "Clinical and biologic prognostic factors in breast cancer diagnosed during postmenopausal hormone replacement therapy." *Obstetrics and Gynecology,* 1995, 85: 11.

Bradlow, H. L., et al. "Indole-3-carbinol: A novel approach to breast cancer prevention." Appearing in "Cancer Prevention. From the Laboratory to the Clinic: Implications of Genetic, Molecular and Preventive Research," *Annals of the New York Academy of Sciences,* September 1995, 768: 180–200. And also: "Multifunctional aspects of the action of indole-3-carbinol as an antitumor agent," *Annals of the New York Academy of Sciences,* 1999, 889: 204–13.

Brody, Jane E. "Restoring ebbing hormones may slow aging." *New York Times,* July 18, 1995, C1.

Brown, N. M., et al. "Prenatal TCDD and predisposition to mammary cancer in the rat." *Carcinogenesis,* September 1998, 19 (9): 1623–9.

Bush, Trudy L. "Preserving cardiovascular benefits of hormone replacement therapy." *Journal of Reproductive Medicine,* March 2000, 45, 3 (Supplement): 259–72.

Buster, J. E., et al. "Postmenopausal steroid replacement with micronized dehydroepiandrosterone: preliminary oral bioavailability and dose proportionality studies," *American Journal of Obstetrics and Gynecology,* 1992, 166: 1163–68.

Carlson, L. E., et al. "Relationships between dehydroepiandrosterone sulfate (DHEAS) and cortisol (CRT) plasma levels and everyday memory in Alzheimer's disease patients compared to healthy controls." *Horm Behav,* June 1999, 35 (3): 254–63.

Cass, Hyla, and McNally, Terrence. *Kava.* Rocklin, Cal.: Prima Publishing, 1998.

Castelo-Branco, C., et al. "Long-term compliance with estrogen replacement therapy in surgical postmenopausal women." *Menopause,* Winter 1999, 6 (4): 307–11.

Cavalieri, E. L., et al., "Molecular origin of cancer: catechol estrogen-3, 4-quinones as endogenous tumor initiators." *Proceedings of the National Academy of Sciences,* September 30, 1997, 94 (20): 10937–42.

Chakmakjian, Z. H., and Zachariah, N. Y. "Bioavailability of progesterone with different modes of administration." *Journal of Reproductive Medicine,* June 1987, 32 (6): 443–47.

Chang, K. J., et al. "Influences of percutaneous administration of estradiol and progesterone on human breast epithelial cell cycle in vivo." *Fertility and Sterility,* April 1995, 63 (4): 785–91.

Claustrat, B., et al. "Melatonin and jet lag: confirmatory result using a simplified protocol." *Biol Psychiatry,* 1992, 32: 705–11.

Colditz, G. A., et al. "Hormone replacement therapy and breast cancer risk." *American Journal of Obstetrics & Gynecology,* 1993, 168: 1473–80.

Collaborative Group on Hormonal Factors in Breast Cancer. "Breast cancer and hormone replacement therapy: Collaborative reanalysis of data from 51 epidemiological studies of 52,705 women with breast cancer and 108,411 women without breast cancer." *Lancet,* 1997, 350: 1047–59.

Cooper, A., et al. "Systemic absorption of progesterone from Progest cream in postmenopausal women." *Lancet,* April 25, 1998, 351 (9111): 1255–6.

Coulan, C. B., et al. "Chronic anovulation may increase postmenopausal breast cancer risk." *Journal of the American Medical Association,* 1983, 249: 445–6.

Cowan, L. D., et al. "Breast cancer incidence in women with a history of progesterone deficiency." *American Journal of Epidemiology,* August 1981, 114 (2): 209–17.

Cromer, B. A. "Effects of hormonal contraceptives on bone mineral density." *Drug Safety,* March 1999, 20 (3): 213–22.

Cundy, T., et al. "Spinal bone density in women using depot medroxyprogesterone contraception." *Obstetrics and Gynecology,* October 1998, 92 (4 pt 1): 569–73.

Davelaer. "Exogenous estrogen (E2) subcutaneous protective?" *Tijdschr Geneeskd,* 1991, 135 (14): 613–15.

Dew, J., et al. "A cohort study of hormonal replacement therapy given to women previously treated for breast cancer." *Climacteric,* 1998, 1: 137–42.

DiSaia, P. J., et al. "Hormone replacement in breast cancer." *Lancet,* 1993, 342: 1232.

———. "Hormone replacement therapy in breast cancer survivors: A cohort study." *American Journal of Obstetrics and Gynecology,* 1996, 174: 1494–98.

Dollins, A. B., et al. "Effect of inducing nocturnal serum melatonin concentrations in daytime on sleep, mood, body temperature, and performance." *Proceedings of the National Academy of Sciences,* 1994, 91: 1824–28.

Eden, J. A., et al. "A case-controlled study of combined continuous estrogen-progestin replacement therapy amongst women with a personal history of breast cancer." *Menopause,* 1995, 2: 67–72.

Ewertz, M. "Influences of noncontraceptive exogenous sex hormones on breast cancer risk in Denmark." Cited by Gambrell, presentation paper.

Feldman, D. L., et al. "Cytoplasmic glucocorticoid binding proteins in bone cells." *Endocrinology,* 1975, 96: 29–36.

Fishman, J., et al. "Increased estrogen-16-alpha-hydroxylase activity in women with breast and endometrial cancer." *Journal of Steroidal Biochemistry,* April 1984, 20 (4B): 1077–81.

Fitzpatrick, Lorraine, and Good, Andrew. "Micronized progesterone: clinical indications and comparison with current treatments." *Fertility and Sterility,* September 1999, 72 (3): 389–97.

Folkard, S., Arendt, J., et al. "Can melatonin improve shift workers' tolerance of the night shift? Some preliminary findings." *Chronobiology Int.,* 1993, 10: 315–20.

Foidart, J., et al. "Estradiol and progesterone regulate the proliferation of human breast epithelial cells." *Fertility and Sterility,* May 1998, 69 (5): 963–68.

Food and Drug Administration. "Tampons and asbestos, dioxin & toxic shock syndrome." Report from the Center for Devices and Radiological Health, July 23, 1999.

Formby, B., and Wiley, T. S. "Progesterone inhibits growth and induces apoptosis in breast cancer cells: inverse effects on Bcl-2 and p53." *Annals of Clinical Laboratory Sci,* November-December 1998, 28 (6): 360–9.

———. "Bcl-2, survivin and variant CD44 v7-v10 are downregulated and p53 is upregulated in breast cancer cells by progesterone: inhibition of cell growth and induction of apoptosis." *Mol Cell Biochem,* December 1999, 202 (1–2): 53–61.

Fortunati, N. "Sex hormone–binding globulin: Not only a transport protein." *Journal of Endocrine Investigation,* March 1999, 22 (3): 223–34.

Franceschi, S., et al. "The role of energy and fat in cancers of the breast and colon-rectum in a southern European population." *Annals of Oncology,* 1999, 10 Supplement 6: 61–3.

Gaby, Alan R. *Preventing and Reversing Osteoporosis.* Rocklin, Cal.: Prima Publications, 1995.

Gajdos, Csaba, et al. "Breast cancer diagnosed during hormone replacement therapy." *Obstetrics and Gynecology,* April 2000, 95 (4): 513–18.

Gambrell, R. Don, et al. "Decreased incidence of breast cancer in postmenopausal estrogen-progestogen users." *Obstetrics-Gynecology,* October 1983, 62 (4):435–43.

Gambrell, R. Don, Jr. "Hormone replacement therapy and breast cancer." *Maturitas,* August 1987, 9 (2): 123–33.

———. "Hormone replacement therapy and breast cancer risk." *Archives of Family Medicine,* June 1996, 5: 341–50.

———. "Breast cancer and HRT." Presentation for medical conference, April 2000.

———. personal communication.

Hargrove, Joel T., et al. "Absorption of oral progesterone is influenced by vehicle and particle size." *American Journal of Obstetrics and Gynecology,* 1989, 161 (4): 948–51.

————. "Menopausal hormone replacement therapy with continuous daily oral micronized estradiol and progesterone." *Obstetrics and Gynecology,* April 1989, 73 (4): 606–12.

Helzlsouer, Kathy, et al. "Relationship of prediagnostic serum levels of dehydroepiandrosterone and dehydroepiandrosterone sulfate to the risk of developing premenopausal breast cancer." *Cancer Research,* January, 1992, 52:1–4.

Holli, K., et al. "Low biologic aggressiveness in breast cancer in women using hormone replacement therapy." *Journal of Clinical Oncology,* 1998, 16: 3115–20.

Holmes, Michelle D., et al. "Association of dietary intake of fat and fatty acids with risk of breast cancer." *Journal of the American Medical Association,* March 10,1999, 281 (10): 914–20.

Hortobagyi, G. I., et al. "Sequential cyclic combined hormonal therapy for metastatic breast cancer." *Cancer,* 1989, 64: 1002–6.

Hulley, S., et al. "Randomized trial of estrogen plus progestin for secondary prevention of coronary heart disease in postmenopausal women. Heart and Estrogen/progestin Replacement Study (HERS) Research Group." *Journal of the American Medical Association,* August 19, 1998, 280 (7): 605–13.

Johannes, C. B., et al. "Relation of dehydroepiandrosterone and dehydroepiandrosterone sulfate with cardiovascular disease risk factors in women: longitudinal results from the Massachusetts Women's Health Study." *Journal of Clinical Epidemiology,* February 1999, 52 (2): 95–103.

Johnson, Kate. "ERT havles testosterone levels, may warrant Tx." *Ob-Gyn News,* May 15, 2000, 35 (10): 18.

Jorgensen, Jens, et al. "Three years of growth hormone treatment in growth hormone-deficient adults: near normalization of body composition and physical performance." *European Journal of Endocrinology,* 1994, 130: 224–8.

Kall, M. A., et al. "Effects of dietary broccoli on human drug metabolising activity." *Cancer Letters,* March 19, 1997, 114 (1–2): 169–70.

Khalsa, Dharma Singh, with Stauth, Cameron. *Brain Longevity.* New York: Warner Books, 1997.

Kidd, Parris. *"Phosphatidylserine."* New Canaan, Conn.: Keats Publishing, 1998.

Klatz, Ronald, and Goldman, Robert. *Stopping the Clock.* New Canaan, Conn.: Keats Publishing, 1996.

Lane, G., et al. "Dose-dependent effects of oral progesterone on the oestro-genised post menopausal endometrium." *British Medical Journal,* 1983, 287: 1241–44.

Lavigne, J. A., et al. "An association between the allele coding for a low activity variant of catechol-O-methyl transferase and the risk for breast cancer." *Cancer Research,* December 15, 1997, 57 (24): 5493–7.

Lee, John R., and Hopkins,Virginia. *What Your Doctor May Not Tell You About Menopause: The Breakthrough Book on Natural Progesterone.* New York: Warner Books, 1996.

Lee, John R. "Women's heart disease, heart attacks, and hormones." *The John R. Lee, MD Medical Letter,* August 1998: 1–3.

———. "Sleep, surviving and breast cancer." *The John R. Lee, MD Medical Letter,* April 2000: 6.

Legros, S., et al. "Premenstrual tension syndrome or premenstrual dysphoria." *Review Med Liege,* April 1999, 54 (4): 268–73.

Leis, H. P., Jr. "Endocrine prophylaxis of breast cancer with cyclic estrogen and progesterone." *International Surgery,* May 1966, 45 (5): 496–503.

Lemon, H. M. "Clinical and experimental aspects of the anti-mammary carinogenic activity of estriol." *Frontier Horm Research,* 1977 (5):155–73.

———. "Pathophysiologic consideration in the treatment of menopausal patients with estrogens: the role of estriol in the prevention of mammary carcinoma." *Acta Endocrinol Suppl (Copenhagen),* 1980, 233: 17–27.

———. "Antimammary carcinogenic activity of 17-alpha-ethinyl estriol." *Cancer,* 1987, 60: 2873–81.

Lemon, H. M., et al. "Inhibition of radiogenic mammary carcinoma in rats by estriol or tamoxifen." *Cancer,* 1989, 63: 1685–92.

Lissoni, P., et al. "Randomized study with the pineal hormone melatonin versus supportive care alone in advanced nonsmall cell lung cancer resistant to a first-line chemotherapy containing cisplatin." *Oncology,* 1992, 49: 336–39.

———. "Decreased toxicity and increased efficacy of cancer chemotherapy using the pineal hormone melatonin in metastatic solid tumor patients with poor clinical status." *European Journal of Cancer,* November 1999, 35 (12): 1688–92.

Lauritzen, C. "Ostrogensubstitution in der postmenopause vor und nach behandeltem genital-und mammakarzinom." *Menopause Hormonsubsitution Heute,* 1993, 6: 76–88.

Magnusson, C., et al. "Prognostic characteristics in breast cancers after hormone replacement therapy." *Breast Cancer Research and Treatment,* 1996, 38: 325–34.

Marsden, J., et al. "Are randomized trials of hormone replacement therapy in symptomatic women with breast cancer feasible?" *Fertility and Sterility,* 2000, 73: 292–99.

Mauvais-Jarvis, P., et al. "Luteal phase defect and breast cancer genesis." *Breast Cancer Research and Treatment,* 1982, 2: 139.

Michnovicz, J. J., and Bradlow, H. L. "Induction of estradiol metabolism by dietary indole-3-carbinole in humans." *Journal of the National Cancer Institute,* June 6, 1990, 82 (11): 947–49.

Miyagawa, K., et al. "Medroxyprogesterone acetate interferes with ovarian steroid protection against coronary vasospasm." *Nature Medicine,* 1997, 3: 324–27.

Mohr, P. E., et al. "Serum progesterone and prognosis in operable breast cancer." *British Journal of Cancer,* June 1996, 73 (12): 1552–55.

Monteleone, P., et al. "Allopregnanolone concentrations and premenstrual syndrome." *European Journal of Endocrinology,* March 2000, 142 (3): 269–73.

Moon, Mary Ann. "HRT users more prone to mammography failures." *Ob-Gyn News,* May 15, 2000, 35 (10): 1.

———. "Breast density predicts mammography failure." *Ob-Gyn News,* May 15, 2000, 35 (10): 15.

Morales, A. J., et al. "Effects of replacement dose of dehydroepiandrosterone in men and women of advancing age." *Journal of Clinical Endocrinology and Metabolism,* 1994, 78 (6): 1360–67.

Mortola, J. F., et al. "The effects of dehydroepiandrosterone on endocrine-metabolic parameters in postmenopausal women." *Journal of Clinical Endocrinology and Metabolism,* 1990, 71: 696–704.

Nachtigall, Lila E. "Emerging delivery systems for estrogen replacement: Aspects of transdermal and oral delivery." *American Journal of Obstetrics and Gynecology,* 1995, 173 (3): 993–97.

Nachtigall, M. J., et al. "Incidence of breast cancer in a 22-year study of women receiving estrogen-progestin replacement therapy." *Obstetrics Gynecology,* 1992, 80: 827–30.

Nafziger, Anne, et al. "Longitudinal changes in dehydroepiandrosterone concentrations in men and women." *Journal of Laboratory Clinical Medicine,* 1998, 131 (4): 316–23.

Natrajan, P. K., Soumakis, K., and Gambrell, R. D. "Estrogen replacement therapy in women with previous breast cancer." *American Journal of Obstetrics and Gynecology,* August 1999, 181 (2): 288–95.

O'Connor, I. F., et al. "Breast carcinoma developing in patients on hormone replacement therapy: a histological and immunohistological study." *Journal of Clinical Pathol,* 1998, 51: 935–38.

Padwick, M. L., et al. "Absorption and metabolism of oral progesterone when administered twice daily." *Fertility & Sterility,* 1986, 46: 402–07.

Persson, I., et al. "Combined oestrogen-progestogen replacement and breast cancer risk." *Lancet,* 1992, 340: 1044.

————. "Risks of breast and endometrial cancer after estrogen and progestin replacement." *Cancer Causes Control,* 1999, 10: 253–60.

Petrie, K., et al. "A double-blind trial of melatonin as a treatment for jet lag in international cabin crew." *Biol Psychiatry,* 1993, 33: 526–30.

Pierpaoli, Walter. "Melatonin, the pineal gland and aging: A planetary and biological reality." In *The Science of Anti-Aging Medicine* (Edited by Klatz and Goldman), Colorado Springs, American Academy of Anti-Aging Medicine, 1996.

Pierpaoli, Walter, and Regelson, William. "The pineal control of aging. The effect of melatonin and pineal grafting on aging mice." *Proceedings of the National Academy of Sciences,* 1994, 91: 787–91.

————. *The Melatonin Miracle.* New York: Pocket Books, 1995.

Plouffe, L., Jr. "Ovaries, androgens and the menopause: practical applications." *Seminars of Reproductive Endocrinology,* 1998, 16 (2): 117–20.

Plu-Bureau, G., et al. "Progestogen use and decreased risk of breast cancer in a cohort study of premenopausal women with benign breast disease." *British Journal of Cancer,* 1994, 70: 270–77.

————. "Percutaneous progesterone use and risk of breast cancer: results from a French cohort study of premenopausal women with benign breast disease." *Cancer Detection and Prevention,* 1999, 23 (4): 290–6.

Powles, T. J., et al. "Hormone replacement therapy after breast cancer." *Lancet,* 1993, 342: 60–61.

Powrie, Jake, et al. "Growth hormone replacement therapy for growth hormone-deficient adults," *Drugs,* 1995, 49 (5): 656–63.

Prior, J. C. "Progesterone as a bone-trophic hormone." *Endocrine Reviews,* May 1990, 11 (2): 386–98.

Raz, Raul, and Stamm, Walter. "A controlled trial of intravaginal estriol in postmenopausal women with recurrent urinary tract infections." *The New England Journal of Medicine,* September 9, 1993, 329 (11): 753–56.

Regelson, William, and Colman, Carol. *The Superhormone Promise: Nature's Antidote to Aging.* New York: Pocket Books, 1997.

Roan, Shari. "Hormone found to raise risk of breast cancer." *Los Angeles Times,* February 7, 2000.

Ron, E., et al. "Cancer incidence in a cohort of infertile women." *American Journal of Epidemiology,* 1987, 125: 780–90.

Rosano, G. M., et al. "Medroxyprogesterone but not natural progesterone reverses the beneficial effect of estradiol-17b upon exercise induced myocardial ischemia: a double-blind cross-over study." *Circulation,* 1996; 94: 1–18.

———. "Cardiovascular pharmacology of hormone replacement therapy." *Drugs & Aging,* September 1999, 15 (3): 219–34.

Rosen, Thord, et al. "Cardiovascular risk factors in adult patients with growth hormone deficiency." *Acta Endocrinologica,* 1993, 129: 195–200.

Rosen, Thord, et al. "Consequences of growth hormone deficiency in adults and the benefits and risks of recombinant human growth hormone treatment," *Hormone Research,* 1995, 43: 93–99.

Ross, R. K., et al. "Effect of hormone replacement therapy on breast cancer risk: estrogen versus estrogen plus progestin." *Journal of the National Cancer Institute,* February 16, 2000, 92 (4): 328–32.

Rupprecht, R., et al. "Neuropsychopharmacological properties of neuroactive steroids." *Steroids,* January-February 1999, 64 (1): 83–91.

Rylance, P. B., et al. "Natural progesterone and antihypertensive action." *British Medical Journal,* January 5, 1985, 290: 13–14.

Salmon, R. J., et al. "Clinical and biological characteristics of breast cancers in postmenopausal women receiving hormone replacement therapy." *Oncology Rep,* 1999, 6: 699–703.

Sarrel, P. M. "Cardiovascular aspects of androgens in women." *Seminars of Reproductive Endocrinology,* 1998, 16 (2): 121–8.

———. "Psychosexual effects of menopause: role of androgens." *American Journal of Obstetrics and Gynecology,* March 1999, 180 (3 pt 2): 319–24.

Sarrel, P. M., et al. "Vasodilator effects of estrogen are not diminished by androgen in postmenopausal women." *Fertility and Sterility,* December 1997, 68 (6): 1125–7.

Schairer, C., Lubin, Jay, et al. "Menopausal estrogen and estrogen-progestin replacement therapy and breast cancer risk." *Journal of the American Medical Association,* January 26, 2000, 283 (4): 485–91.

Seelig, Mildred. "Interrelationship of magnesium and estrogen in cardiovascular and bone disorders, eclampsia, and premenstrual syndrome." *Journal of the American College of Nutrition,* 1993, 12 (4): 442–58.

Senie, R. T., et al. "Timing of breast cancer excision during the menstrual cycle and influences duration of disease-free survival." *Annals of Internal Medicine,* 1991, 115: 337–42.

———. "The timing of breast cancer surgery during the menstrual cycle." *Oncology,* October 1997, 11 (10): 1509–17.

Service, Robert F. "New role for estrogen in cancer?" *Science,* March 13, 1998, 279: 1631–33.

Shaywitz, Sally, et al. "Effects of estrogen on brain activation patterns in postmenopausal women during working memory tasks." *Journal of the American Medical Association,* 1999, 281: 1197–1202.

Sherwin, B. B. "The impact of different doses of estrogen and progestin on mood and sexual behavior in postmenopausal women." *Journal of Clinical Endocrinology and Metabolism,* February 1991, 72 (2): 336–43.

———. "Sex hormones and psychological functioning in postmenopausal women." *Exp Gerontol,* 1994, 29 (3–4): 423–30.

———. "Can estrogen keep you smart? Evidence from clinical studies." *Journal of Psychiatry Neuroscience,* September 1999, 24 (4): 315–21.

Shimada, T., et al. "Activation of chemically diverse procarcinogens by human cytochrome P-450 1B1." *Cancer Research,* July 1996, 56 (13): 2979–84.

Siegal, Sanford. *Is Your Thyroid Making You Fat?* New York: Warner Books, 2000.

Smith, Sheryl, et al. "GABA receptor alpha4 subunit suppression prevents withdrawal properties of an endogenous steroid." *Nature,* 1998, 392: 926–30.

Speroff, Leon. "Postmenopausal estrogen-progestin therapy and breast cancer: a clinical response to an epidemiological report." *Contemporary Ob/Gyn,* March 2000: 103–121.

Stanford, J. L., Weiss, N. S., et al. "Combined estrogen and progestin hormone replacement therapy in relation to risk of breast cancer in middle-aged women." *Journal of the American Medical Association,* 2000, 283: 485–91.

Steenland, Kyle, et al. "Cancer, heart disease, and diabetes in workers exposed to 2, 3, 7, 8-tetrachlorodibenzo-p-dioxin." *Journal of the National Cancer Institute,* May 5, 1999, 91(9): 779–86.

Taylor, Maida. "Alternatives to conventional hormone replacement therapy." *Comprehensive Therapy,* 1997, 23 (8): 514–32.

Vaccarino, V., et al. "Sex-based differences in early mortality after myocardial infarction." *New England Journal of Medicine,* July 22, 1999, 341 (4): 217–25.

VanVollenhoven, R. F., et al. "An open study of dehydroepiandrosterone in systemic lupus erythematosus." *Arthritis Rheum,* 1994, 37: 1305–10.

Wagner, Janice. "Rationale for hormone replacement therapy in atherosclerosis prevention." *The Journal of Reproductive Medicine,* March 2000, 45 (3 Supplement): 245–58.

———. "Cardiovascular considerations for hormone replacement therapy." *International Journal of Fertility,* March 2000, 45 (Supplement 1): 73–80.

Wallis, Claudia. "The estrogen dilemma." *Time,* June 26, 1995. Cover article.

Watts, N. B., et al. "Comparison of oral estrogens and estrogens plus androgen on bone mineral density, menopausal symptoms, and lipid-lipoprotein profiles in surgical menopause." *Obstetrics and Gynecology,* April 1995, 85 (4): 529–37.

Welty, F. K. "Who should receive hormone replacement therapy?" *Journal of Thrombolysis,* 1996, 3 (1): 13–21.

Wexler, Laura. "Studies of acute coronary syndromes in women—Lessons for everyone." *New England Journal of Medicine,* July 22, 1999, 341 (4): 275–6.

Wile, A. G., et al. "Hormone replacement therapy in previously treated breast cancer patients." *American Journal of Surgery,* 1993, 165: 372–75.

Williams, Timothy, and Frohman, Lawrence. "Potential therapeutic indications for growth hormone–releasing hormone in conditions other than growth retardation." *Pharmacotherapy,* November/December 1986, 6 (6): 311–16.

Willett, Walter. "Dietary fat and breast cancer." *Toxicol Sciences,* December 1999, 52 (2 Supplement): 127–46.

Willett, Walter, et al. "Postmenopausal estrogens—opposed, unopposed, or none of the above." *Journal of the American Medical Association,* January 26, 2000, 283, (4): 534–5.

Willis, Dawn, et al. "Estrogen replacement therapy and risk of fatal breast cancer in a prospective cohort of postmenopausal women in the United States." *Cancer Causes Control,* July 1996, 8 (4): 672.

Wright, Jonathan V., and Morgenthaler, John. *Natural Hormone Replacement.* Petaluma, Cal.: Smart Publications, 1997.

Yen, S. S., et al. "Replacement of DHEA in aging men and women. Potential remedial effects." *Annals of the New York Academy of Sciences,* 1995, 774: 128–42.

Zinder, O., et al. "Neuroactive steroids: their mechanism of action and their function in the stress response." *Acta Physiol Scand,* November 1999, 167 (3): 181–8.

Acknowledgments

The authors wish to express their gratitude to the following individuals:

Yfat Reiss, for her enthusiasm and winning suggestions.

Richard Fura, of Kronos Compounding Pharmacy in Las Vegas, and Wally Simons of Women's International Pharmacy of Madison, Wisconsin, and Sun City West, Arizona, for providing practical information on compounding pharmacies and, above all, for the consistently high quality of natural hormones they have provided to my patients over the years.

Mitchell Ivers, our editor at Pocket Books, for his encouragement, support, and skilled editorial guidance.

Jack Scovil, a superb agent and advisor.

Doctors Ronald Klatz and Bob Goldman for their vision to create a dynamic new medical organization—The American Academy of Anti-Aging Medicine—dedicated to helping maximize both quality and quantity of life.

Index

About the Authors

Obstetrician-gynecologist and antiaging specialist Uzzi Reiss, M.D., has been a leader in the clinical application of natural hormones, nutrition, mind/body principles, and other innovative methods. While serving free clinics in New York and Los Angeles at the start of his career, up to the present day, in his highly successful Beverly Hills practice, he has used these approaches to optimize the health of many thousands of patients. In 1997, Reiss opened the Beverly Hills Anti-Aging Center as a natural expansion of his prevention-oriented practice. He is one of the first medical doctors in the United States to become board-certified by the American Academy of Anti-Aging Medicine. The Israeli-born physician earned his medical degree at the Technion Institute of Technology in Haifa and completed his U.S. residency in obstetrics and gynecology at the Albert Einstein College of Medicine in New York. Visit Dr. Reiss's Web site at www.naturalhormonebalance.net for updates on hormonal information and case histories.

Coauthor Martin Zucker has written extensively on natural healing, nutrition, fitness, and alternative medicine for more than twenty years. Zucker is a former newsman and correspondent for Associated Press in Europe and the Middle East. He has coauthored or ghostwritten ten books, including *The Miracle of MSM—The Natural Solution for Pain* (G. P. Putnam's Sons, 1999). He is a contributing editor to *Let's Live*, one of the country's oldest preventive medicine publications.

Zucker's relationship with Dr. Reiss goes back nearly twenty years. He first wrote about Reiss's innovative gynecological treatments in the early 1980s. On a personal note, Reiss has delivered five of Zucker's six grandchildren.